Practical Ways to Better Mental Health
Food and Lifestyle Strategies

I0555089

ISBN
979-8-21814-454-8 Paperback

This book is dedicated to my father who passed away at 91 years of age, while I was still in the process of writing it. Throughout his life, my dad ate well, exercised daily, and kept his mind active. I will remember him as a man who had incredible strength, unwavering perseverance, and steadfast faith in God, and lived his life with dignity and humility.

Table of Contents

Preface...1

Introduction...4

Chapter 1: About Mental Health....................................9

Chapter 2: The Gut-Brain Connection.........................24

Chapter 3: The Role of Nutrition in Mental Health....28

Chapter 4: Foods and Supplements to Support Mental Health....38

Chapter 5: Therapies for Better Mental Health...........56

Chapter 6: Genetics..67

Conclusion..73

Appendix A: How to Choose Quality Supplements.....................75

Appendix B: Food and Mood Journal...76

Glossary...77

Index..80

Acknowledgements...86

About the Author...88

Endnotes..89

Preface

It was January 2014 when I realized that the vicious cycle of anxious thoughts and feelings I was experiencing might not ever end. I remember that moment as if it were yesterday. My anxiety levels were increasing even though I wasn't experiencing any particularly stressful situations in my life at the time.

Twice in one month that year, I made trips to the hospital emergency room because I experienced alarming sensations – my heart felt like it was beating out of my chest. I wondered if I was having a heart attack. On both my trips to the ER, my blood pressure was off the charts, and I had an extremely rapid heart rate. The ER doctor instructed the nurses to monitor my blood pressure and heart rate continuously and to draw blood to run tests. I was not discharged until my blood pressure and heart rate reached an acceptable range.

When you leave the ER, the paperwork given to the patient always recommends a follow up visit with your primary care physician. In my case it was also recommended that I follow up with a cardiologist. After my appointment with the cardiologist, I was told there was nothing wrong with my heart. However, I was diagnosed with primary hypertension. After my ER visit and the cardiologist visit, my primary care physician diagnosed me with a generalized anxiety disorder. All I could ask myself was "what is that"? I knew nothing about anxiety disorders and my primary care physician provided very little information to explain this condition. However, she did prescribe anti-anxiety and blood pressure lowering medications.

Just after I was diagnosed, I started researching generalized anxiety disorder and found that it is classified as a mental health disorder. Typical treatment for someone with this disorder is medication and therapy. I can't say which treatment option would have been the best choice for me because I did not have enough background information in this area. Mental health issues were never discussed in my family—I would have been considered "weak" if I hinted about suffering from anything related to anxiety or depression. In my culture, I was taught to work hard, push through it, deal with it, and to find strength in my faith. As the anxiety ebbed and flowed, I felt like a failure in life. As a Christian, I questioned my faith in God. After all, I've been taught that I am supposed to live in peace and not worry.

Weeks after the initial episode, I started experiencing even more anxiety, as well as mild depression. I slept on the sofa in my home office because this was my "safe place." I worked from home because I was too anxious to have human interaction. I had reached a point where the usual daily activities, like grocery shopping, driving, or spending time with friends, were challenging. I always had this feeling of impending doom as if I were going to die. I sat and cried and for no reason. As my mental health deteriorated, so did my physical health. I had very little appetite, lost ten pounds, and experienced excruciating neck and shoulder pain. These symptoms lasted for weeks. Anxiety and depression had taken control of my life. I never took the anti-anxiety medication, and I chose not to share my anguish with anyone. My husband was worried and confused about my physical and mental health and thought it was related to menopause. My children thought I was just being "mom" getting older and a little eccentric.

For months, I suffered in silence as I became increasingly fearful. I bottled up my problems in hopes that my family, friends, and other people would not notice. Perhaps worst of all, I no longer saw myself as a strong woman like my mother, grandmother, and aunts who were "superwomen" and could "keep on keeping on" despite their circumstances. This was a very dangerous period in my life because I placed my mental and physical health at risk by effectively ignoring the problem.

It has taken me years to talk openly and without shame about my anxiety. Through this experience, I learned what steps I needed to take to address my mental health disorder. These steps included acknowledging that I had a mental health problem, documenting the symptoms, and talking with a trained professional. It took me a while to realize that there was no reason to be ashamed. Later, I was surprised to learn that anxiety disorders are the most common health disorder in the United States, and impact many women who, just like me, keep silent about their condition.

My experiences and my personal research encouraged me to pursue a healthy body and a healthy mind. If I'm fortunate enough to live to a ripe old age, I hope that my mind continues to function well, even if my physical body starts failing. Of course, I want to do what I can to protect my physical health, but I now know that there are things I can do to protect my mental health as well. There are many other people like me who struggle with mental health issues which they try to hide or suppress. I wrote this book so every reader will have the basic information describing mental health disorders and knowledge of various foods and therapies to combat them. Ultimately, I want to encourage anyone who struggles with these types of issues to seek the help they need.

Please be advised that the specific nutrition suggestions, therapies, and interventions presented in this book may not be the best approach for some individuals and should not replace your current medications and/or any professional therapy that you are receiving. If you are struggling with a mental health disorder, it's important to seek professional help. Seeking help doesn't make you weak; it makes you wise.

Introduction

"Anxiety happens when you think you have to figure out everything all at once. Breathe. You're strong. You got this. Take it day by day."

– Karen Salmansohn

Do you struggle sometimes to talk about your mental health, or engage in a conversation with someone else about mental health? If so, I want you to know that you are not alone. Many of us are embarrassed or ashamed to talk about this seemingly sensitive issue. What if you were having problems with your heart or liver and had to take medication to correct that problem? — would you be ashamed or embarrassed? Probably not because there usually isn't stigma associated with treating medical issues. So, why is it that if your brain stops functioning correctly, there is a stigma? A mental health disorder is not a sign of weakness and requires attention and intervention just as a physical health disorder does. The struggle is real and should be taken seriously.

Making the decision to honestly address your mental health may not be easy, but is empowering. Time and time again, people who are seeking treatment for mental health disorders feel the stigma associated with treatment such as therapy. I have heard many people say, "I don't need to see a therapist because I'm not crazy." And if they are seeing a therapist, they don't want to publicize the fact. Nevertheless, it is vital that we start to speak openly about these disorders, without stigma, judgment, or shame. This is especially important in our homes, workplaces, and communities. In recent years, mental health issues have increased and some conversations about mental health have come into focus in the public realm. For instance, sports figures Simone Biles, a USA Olympic gymnast, Noemi Osaka, a top tennis player, and Michael Phelps, an Olympic swimmer, along with other well-known athletes, have spoken out publicly about their struggles with their mental health issues.

It's not just athletes who struggle with mental health issues. People of all professions may find themselves battling these same mental health disorders. Physicians, nurses, journalists, judges, lawyers, pastors, musicians, teachers, truck drivers, cooks, students, housewives, and retirees can all be affected. The Bible even documents men and women of great faith from thousands of years ago facing these struggles. Although the Bible does not use the words "mental health", it is referred to by similar words such as "brokenhearted", "troubled", and "downcast." Job, one of the many great men of courage of the Bible, suffered an enormous tragedy which caused him to become mentally and physically ill. He says, "I have no peace, no quietness, I have no rest, but only turmoil" (Job 3:26), and "Terrors overwhelm me … and now my life ebbs away; days of suffering grip me. Night pierces my bones, my gnawing pains never rest" (Job 30:15-17). Hannah experienced depression when she was harassed by her husband's other wife. She stated, "…she provoked her; therefore she wept and did not eat" (1 Samuel 1:7).

The truth is our mental health and physical health are more connected than we realize. Many of us get annual physical exams or health screenings for various possible illnesses and focus on looking good and staying fit. Yet, we do not take the same proactive approach towards our mental health. Many years ago, a coworker told me he was "taking a mental health day off." I imagined that he was escaping a day of work to "play hooky." But now I know better. There are times when we need to step away from our work, responsibilities, or routine to take care of our mental state and prevent a possible downward spiral. For some people, this may mean a day of extra rest, but for others it may be a day to "have fun."

Understanding mental health is more important than ever. The World Health Organization (WHO) states that "Mental health is a state of well-being in which an individual realizes his or her own abilities, can cope with the normal stresses of life, can work productively and is able to make a contribution to his or her community." Mood and anxiety disorders are drastically increasing and even more so since the COVID-19 pandemic due to the virus, lockdowns, isolation, less in-person socializing, more time using social media, and unhealthy eating. According to the Substance Abuse and Mental Health Services Administration, in 2020 about one in five adults in the United States live with a mental health disorder, with a degree of severity ranging from mild to severe. Anxiety disorders affect more than 40 million Americans. Depression affects one in ten and is growing at an alarming rate. Mental health disorders are major factors affecting our health without regard to age, race, gender, and ethnicity. According to the Anxiety and Depression Association of America, people with anxiety disorders go to the doctor three times more frequently than the general population. Disorders like anxiety and depression have been associated with increased risk for developing heart disease, stroke, high blood pressure, type 2 diabetes, stomach ulcers, sleep problems, and other conditions. And most alarming is that the anxiety and depression rates are rising among children and teens. It's not hard to see why if we consider social media. Negative reactions and comments to posts can be very upsetting for all of us. Whether you are a child, teen, adult, or senior, a struggle with any type of mental disorder can disrupt your life. It's important to understand that not everyone will experience a mental health disorder, but everyone will experience periods of time when they struggle with their mental health, just as we all have some physical health challenges at one time or another.

The signs and symptoms of a potential mental health disorder vary from person to person. Recognizing the signs is not always obvious or easy to spot. After all, the phrase "I am fine" is often our favorite response to the "How are you" question. Right? Some common signs of a mental health disorder include increased hunger, lack of appetite, feeling excessively sad, excessive worrying, mood changes, avoiding friends, and avoiding social activities. What many people may not realize is that all these symptoms may also be the result of our dietary choices. In recent years researchers have shown how food can influence our mental health. This is known as nutritional psychiatry. Another area of science called nutrigenomics is revealing how the foods we eat help us adapt and optimize our health based on our genetic blueprint. This book will provide you with a basic understanding of mental health, a detailed description of the role nutrition plays in mental health, and an explanation of how the bacteria (or the microbiome) in our gut can influence our mental health. I also provide information detailing both nutritious foods that can potentially help manage mental health disorder symptoms, as well as problematic foods that are best avoided. In the following chapters I will show you how nutrition, nutritional psychiatry, nutrigenomics, and other approaches such as regular exercise and cooking, all directly and indirectly, play a role in your mental health.

At this point you may be wondering, why would a nutritionist care so much about mental health, and shouldn't she stick to nutrition advice? I wrote this book because I strongly believe many mental health issues can get better by improving your diet. What you eat matters. The information presented in this book is backed by evidence-based scientific research and my personal experience demonstrating the impact of nutrition on mental health. You will be reading about ideas for change in diet and a variety of strategies that you can try based on personal preference and effectiveness. The more we talk about mental health, the more acceptable it will be for those suffering from mental health disorders. Food provides opportunity for connections. There are psychological benefits associated with preparing and enjoying meals with others. Whether we are at a family barbeque, a Sunday night dinner, or at a restaurant enjoying a meal with family and friends, the gathering is an environment for sharing. It is my vision as a nutritionist, that we begin to normalize the conversation around nutrition and its connection to mental health. My hope is that this book will provide motivation to get a conversation started.

Please be advised that the specific nutrition suggestions and interventions presented in this book may not be the best approach for some individuals and should not replace your current medications and/or any professional therapy you are currently receiving. If you are struggling with a mental health disorder, it's important to seek the help you need. Seeking help doesn't make you weak; it makes you wise.

CHAPTER ONE

ABOUT MENTAL HEALTH

"When we are no longer able to change a situation, we are challenged to change ourselves."

— Viktor E. Frankl, Man's Search for Meaning

Remember the song "Don't worry, be happy" by Bobby McFarrin? As simple as this statement may sound, it is probably the last thing someone struggling with their mental health wants to hear. This is especially true for those of us who are frequently anxious or sad. Occasional anxiety and depression are common, but chronic feelings of worry, fear and hopelessness are not. When persistent worry about the future or the past gets out of hand, a wide range of mental health disorders such as anxiety, depression or other psychological issues can follow.

Often, many people use blanket terms such as anxiety, depression, sadness, and suicidal thoughts to describe mental health. But mental health is much more than that. Mental health involves emotions, attitudes, and behaviors. It is something we all have and is part of being human. According to Dr. Daniel Amen, America's leading psychiatrist and brain health expert, mental health is the "ability to use your brain and mind to create the life you want." Our mental health is important because it impacts how we feel, behave, make decisions, cope with stress and other negative life events, and connect to others.

When we fail to address our mental health, we can develop long-standing consequences and worsening of symptoms as we age.

How we respond to different stressors and life circumstances affects our mental health and those responses can move along a mental health intensity spectrum as shown in Figure 1. There are various mental and physical symptoms (e.g., headaches, fatigue, heart palpitations, dizziness) that can occur within this mental health spectrum which can be mild, moderate, or severe in intensity. You can be at one end of the spectrum today, and be at the other end of the spectrum next week. You may also just be languishing somewhere in the middle and not show signs of a mental health disorder. You may just feel "blah" – you are neither happy nor sad. Mental health disorders may be comprised of more than one symptom, may not be linear, and can last for a short time, or be long term. For example, anxiety over the next day's activities, work problems, or one's own physical health can last for a few days without any recognizable symptoms. But anxiety can also escalate and lead to a full-blown panic attack. The changes in intensity can be very frightening to experience.

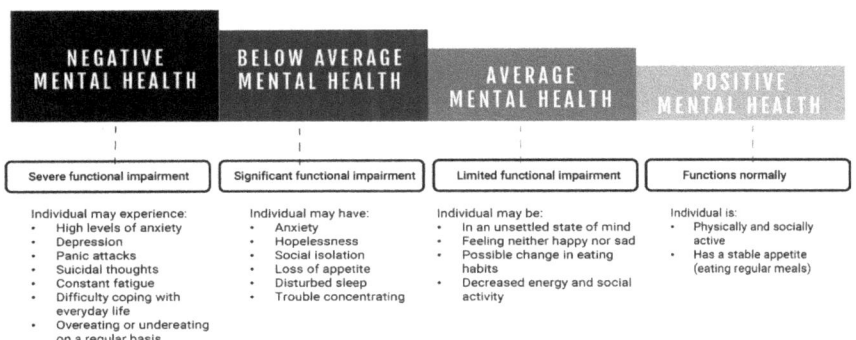

Figure 1: Mental Health Intensity Spectrum

There are many different types of mental health disorders, each of which can change an individual's behavior, thoughts, and feelings in some way. Depression, anxiety, panic disorder, bipolar disorder, and schizophrenia are all examples that can have great impact on life. This chapter will focus mainly on anxiety and depression. The cause of most mental health disorders involves a complex combination of factors which include poor diet (such as excessive amounts of sugar or processed foods), trauma, negative life events, fear, financial struggles, loneliness, isolation, poverty, chronic stress, drug or alcohol abuse, genetic predispositions, nutritional deficiencies, hormonal imbalances, thyroid issues, and personality. People suffering from a mental health disorder typically have a combination of issues contributing to the problem. For example, drug and alcohol abuse commonly occurs in conjunction with mental health disorders. The drugs and/or alcohol are used to ease the mental health symptoms, but have the opposite effect, making symptoms more pronounced and inevitably more difficult to cope with when not using these substances.

With all this in mind, let's turn our attention to two of the most common mental health disorders affecting Americans: anxiety and depression. These two disorders have a lot in common in that they are related psychologically, involve negative thoughts, and share physical symptoms such as nausea, headaches, and digestive problems. The major difference between the two disorders, is that anxiety is characterized by nervous feelings, apprehension, and persistent worry about the future and the past. Individuals with anxiety often dwell obsessively on the past and/or worry excessively about the future. Instead of living in the present which they can control, they may "feel stuck" in the past, which cannot be changed, or "immobilized" by the future, which has yet to happen. Depression, on the other hand, does not usually involve debilitating fear, but is centered around a sense of hopelessness. It is not uncommon for someone to suffer from both anxiety and depression at the same time.

Anxiety

> *"I recall being in 6th grade one evening, watching "Little House on the Prairie" in our basement (since my parents were not TV people they finally capitulated and got us a small black and white TV which they placed in the basement to discourage excessive watching), and I was overcome with this sensation I now know as anxiety. I never had experienced this before. I remember the skirt I was wearing, the chair I was sitting in, and I remember looking down at my skinny freckled legs feeling like something*

was just "off" and it was so unsettling. I couldn't put my finger on it. I just knew it was an unfamiliar feeling, seemed to come out of the blue, and I felt very uncomfortable, like I couldn't "shake it." I now know I had a flood of adrenaline and cortisol and that was part of the physical discomfort, and it was so unlike anything I had felt before that it was etched in my brain." - Sarah

Sometimes the onset of anxiety can be linked to a particular event. Sarah's story illustrates the sudden occurrence of anxiety without any apparent trigger. The next story shows how anxiety, triggered by a fear of flying, affected Trevor's mental state as a child and adolescent.

"The earliest time I can recall feeling what I now understand as anxiety, was around the age of 12. I had emotions that could be construed as nervous energy, general sadness, or seasonal depression prior to this, but I am entirely unsure if I was cognizant of these emotions until the flight. My family and I were on our way to visit some relatives on the east coast. People were still shuffling into further sections of the plane. Suddenly, immense waves of terror set in from seemingly nowhere. I could not breathe. I never had such an intensely negative sensation. I can remember the thought process of having no escape, unable to have control of where I was oriented and lacking access to "fresh air." At that time, I never shared this with anyone because I was ashamed. As a Black male I was taught to act tough and avoid emotional expression. In the years to follow I would sleep a lot during the daytime to ease the symptoms associated with my anxiety. Much of my young adolescence years were spent processing how much this moment affected my reactions to new, uncomfortable, and challenging situations as an adult. However, the anxiety and depression I experience today is much milder. Needless to say, my mental health state is constantly changing." - Trevor

Trevor did not realize that occasional feelings of anxiety and depression are natural. Unfortunately, mental health education is often overlooked both in schools and in our homes. But, basic knowledge in this area can be a critical life skill for all of us. Parents and caregivers should have a basic understanding of mental health so that they can talk to their children about it. Schools should include mental health in the instruction regarding overall health. The importance of proper nutrition as it relates to mental well-being should be part of these discussions.

Anxiety is a word that is often used casually today, but means different things to different people. Many people use the term to describe feelings of endless worry. And anxiety certainly includes worrying. Corrie ten Boom, Christian writer, and public speaker, describes worry as "a cycle of inefficient thoughts whirling around the center of fear." Anxiety can be characterized by excessive nervous feelings, apprehension, and worry about some future event. But this term also can be used to describe normal feelings individuals have when they are stressed, in danger or threatened.

It is normal to have some anxiety in certain circumstances, such as when giving a presentation or speaking in front of others, starting a new job, going on a first date, or confronting a frightening situation. This type of anxiety can even be "healthy" when facing an experience in which you feel some discomfort. Sometimes anxious moments help us make sound decisions, like riding a motorcycle with a helmet to prevent the risk of head injury. As we successfully navigate these types of events in which we experience some level of anxiety, we then develop increased confidence that can help us face future circumstances which may evoke feelings of fear.

When we are in an anxious moment, the normal response for our body is to initiate a flight or fight response. The powerful hormone responsible for this action is called cortisol; it is released when we are under stress, and it triggers a cascade of physiological changes like increased heart rate and blood pressure, and the brain's use of glucose, all which help us to survive an immediate threat. However, for people with an anxiety disorder, this adaptive strategy becomes detrimental. Here are some examples of anxiety that might be spiraling out of control: having persistent and excessive fear and apprehension that overwhelms your thoughts (like the fear of getting sick); expecting a worst-case scenario; always feeling like your brain is on "high-alert"; inability to handle uncertainty about the present moment, and about how life will play out in the future. These internal thought struggles can cause intense physical reactions and may interfere with the ability to deal with everyday activities. When dealing with anxiety, even simple tasks like making a phone call or sending an email may overwhelm you.

Anxiety disorders are one of the most common mental health disorders in the United States today, affecting over 40 million adults over 18 years of age. There are several types of anxiety disorders which include panic disorder, social anxiety disorder, Generalized Anxiety Disorder (GAD), Post Traumatic Stress Disorder (PTSD), Obsessive-Compulsive Disorder (OCD), illness anxiety disorder (also called hypochondria) and various phobias (such as social phobia or claustrophobia). This is not an exhaustive list of anxiety disorders, but covers the most common conditions. According to the Diagnostic and Statistical Manual (DSM-5), GAD is described as "Excessive anxiety and worry (apprehensive expectation), occurring more days than not for at least 6 months, about a number of events or activities (such as work or school performance)." Each type of anxiety disorder is different. Some people with GAD, like me, have constant worry, which sometimes occurs for no apparent reason. These types of anxiety disorders may originate from various risk factors such as improper diet, lack of sleep, low blood sugar, hormonal imbalances, genetic factors, and negative life events or trauma.

Here is a story of a woman who describes an anxious and traumatic episode that occurred when she was a young adult:

> *"I hated high school. I did anything to avoid being there. I always felt on edge, unsafe, and like I didn't belong there. I didn't like too many of the people. I didn't have too many friends as most everyone partied, drank, and did drugs which was most certainly not my thing. I did have a boyfriend who became my best friend. He helped school feel tolerable and safe most days. My boyfriend would always meet me at my locker between 5th and 6th period, but on this Wednesday afternoon he did not show up. I felt a little uneasy, but I thought maybe he got out of his last period class late. During class I kept constantly checking*

my phone and mid-way through 6th period of American history I got a text from a friend who worked in the office who said my boyfriend was in the assistant principal's office. Word spread quickly that he got caught with drugs. Panic ensued over me, I remember getting hot and sweaty, and like I couldn't breathe. I got out of class and felt paralyzed. I essentially blacked out at this point and didn't remember much. I didn't know how to feel. I was scared and anxious all at the same time. Today, I am still dealing with this very adverse event."- Marianne

Author and spiritual teacher, Eckhart Tolle, uses the concept of "painbody" or an old emotional pain that is living inside the body to help us get a better understanding of the trauma experienced by this woman. He explains that past traumatic experiences are persistent because these painful experiences were not completely accepted in the moment in which they occurred. When we have lived through negative and potentially devastating life experiences we generally hold on to our fears and their stressful memories which then compromise our mental health. According to Dr. Bruce Perry, psychiatrist and trauma expert, "childhood adversity or trauma plays a role in 45% of all childhood mental health disorders and 30% of mental health disorders among adults." Other studies that confirm these estimates show that unresolved traumatic childhood experiences can severely impact our health, life, and relationships, which can increase the risk for depression, anxiety, and other mental health disorders.

Although there are different types of anxiety disorders, common physical signs and symptoms may include: sleep problems, loss of appetite, low mood, lightheadedness, agitation, and digestive issues. Other physical symptoms also associated with anxiety disorders include shortness of breath, racing heart, sweating, restlessness, fatigue, headache, muscle tension, difficulty swallowing, and frequent urination. Emotional or behavioral symptoms may include intrusive thoughts, or excessive worrying about potential threat or catastrophe, inability to concentrate on things that matter to you, disinterest in meeting new friends, preoccupation with serious illness, and frequently postponing activities. There are times when a person may suffer from these symptoms, but no one notices. It can be hard to spot the anxiety disorder. This is especially true if the individual appears successful and coping well in life. In reality, this person may be dealing with high levels of anxiety and dealing with fear.

There are so many things in life that can escalate our anxiety levels. Examples of common anxiety triggers include specific foods we eat (such as too much caffeine during the day or close to bedtime), pressure from friends and family who may be testing your patience, high demands at your job, medications, spending lots of time on social media platforms, medical disorders, and menopause. This young female struggled with a lot of anxiety when her parents divorced when she was 15 years of age:

> *"I struggled with anxiety when my parents divorced and a little while after that. Sometimes I'd have panic attacks that would make me just fling myself outside to suck in fresh air. Or if I was driving, I'd turn the air conditioner on high or I'd roll all the windows down. What triggered my anxiety when I was younger was not having the family unit that I was used to having. I was very shy, and I stuck close to both parents so them not being together anymore broke something apart in me and I feared what that would do. In those days I remember my mom taking me to the doctor a few times because I would get so nervous, I wouldn't eat, which caused me to lose weight. With a nervous stomach, everything I ate would make me sick. When the doctor asked me what was going on I said my parents are divorcing. I can remember my mom crying after seeing me cry in the doctor's office. Once they did divorce, I busied myself as best as I could and tried to reset my life. My anxiety these days is a lot different than when I was younger. It's more related to life experiences that I haven't had yet, thinking that I'm running out of time when I let it get to me, or having a shortfall of money, living paycheck to paycheck."- Sabrina*

Another anxiety trigger to consider is TV news. The International Journal of Behavioral Medicine cited a study that showed an increase in anxiety after people watched 15 minutes of television news. And what was alarming was even after distracting the participants with other activities, they were not able to return to their baseline emotional level that was recorded before they started watching the news. This news can negatively impact your mental health over the long-term. I'm not suggesting you stop watching news or stay uninformed regarding local, country, or world events. However, if you are someone who turns on the TV subconsciously or compulsively throughout the day and you find yourself becoming anxious, stressed, or saddened by the sensationalized information, then it may be best to limit your exposure to the news to specific times of the day, perhaps midday.

Other anxiety triggers could be worry about your own health, stress over the next day's activity, and financial pressures. One trigger for my anxiety is using "Doctor Google" to diagnose a condition or disease for various physical symptoms that I am experiencing or researching the meaning of various blood test results. As if the internet was not enough to worsen our anxious thoughts, we sometimes find other creative ways to stress over our ailments. A friend told me that before the invention of internet she would try to find the answers for all her symptoms by first looking in her parent's medical book at home. If she did not find what she was looking for, she would then go the local bookstore where she would spend hours leafing through medical books.

Most of us who deal with an anxiety disorder do not realize that it can do all the following: increase the risk for blood pressure leading to heart disease, cause depression, and initiate the development of other anxiety disorders. Heart disease pertains to various conditions that can affect the heart and blood flow to the heart such as coronary artery disease and heart failure. When you are suffering from constant anxiety for extended periods, your body begins to change. There is reduced blood flow to the heart, increased heart rate, increased blood pressure, and elevated cortisol, the hormone that is released when we are under chronic stress. Eventually, these physiological changes can lead to heart disease. An example of a physical manifestation that recently affected me was worsening of the grinding and clenching of my teeth weeks after my father's untimely death. This caused my temporomandibular joint or TMJ (the hinge that connects your jaw to your skull) to become irritated and painful. I was unaware of the impact that the pent-up anxiety and internalization of my emotions was having on my physical health. Here is a story shared by a friend who had a similar experience about the physical effects resulting from her anxiety disorder:

> *"My body experiences anxiety at night while I am asleep. Not only do I clench my jaw tightly, but I also have restless leg syndrome which I don't usually experience during the day, but my legs start shaking as if I'm having a seizure while I'm asleep! My partner often wakes up thinking there is an earthquake. I think it's all connected and sometimes I carry over feelings during the day. It's a cycle: stress and anxiety cause pain (in this case jaw pain from clenching) and then I experience more anxiety because I have the pain. I often go months without feeling impacted by this, but I do notice flare ups during particularly stressful times in my life."*   - Nikki

Depression

When I was in high school, I was required to read Charlotte Perkins Gilman's short story *The Yellow Wallpaper* in my English literature class. The story was about a woman who after giving birth, battles with postpartum depression, which was called at that time "slight hysterical tendency." The cure for her ailment was to rest, stay indoors, do no work, and refrain from participation in social gatherings. In the end, the woman never left her room that was covered with yellow wallpaper. She envisioned herself as a part of the wallpaper. The wallpaper had become her only stimulant in this secluded environment. Today and especially during the COVID-19 pandemic, many of us are battling mental health issues just like this woman. Oftentimes we are labeled as crazy, eccentric, psychotic, and even out of control. This story is a reminder of how depression is more than just feeling sad, and how debilitating it can be.

Depression is a very complex disorder and there are several types. Some of the most common ones are major depressive disorder, postpartum depression, Seasonal Affective Disorder (SAD), bipolar disorder, and atypical depression. Depression is characterized by extreme sadness that can last for days, months or years

The underlying causes of depression are not fully understood, but research shows that it may be influenced by a combination of many different factors including poor food choices, unhealthy lifestyle habits, inflammation, hormone imbalance, nutritional needs, genetics, and increased alcohol and drug consumption. Other risk factors include family history of depression, excessive social media use, having a chronic disease such as cancer, feelings of rejection, and major life changes such as divorce or death of a loved one. But some depressive episodes can start without any external causes. According to the National Alliance on Mental Illness, approximately one in five adults experiences mental illness in any given year. In 2019, almost 5% of US adults aged 18 and over had regular feelings of depression.

In the following case, this female relative struggled with depression after the death of a child:

> *"I've struggled with depression longer than I probably care to admit. But one of my deepest depression episodes occurred as a result of the death of my first child. He was born with cerebral palsy and was a paraplegic. I knew he wouldn't live a long life, but when he died, I sank into a state of depression that took months to find my way out of that dark time. My state of mind during that time was full of sadness and deep-rooted loneliness. Though there was plenty of support around me, I kept all my feelings to myself, and didn't – or wouldn't, let anyone in. As a family, we never talked about our feelings, so keeping them inside and struggling with the severity of it, seemed natural to some degree. The light shone into my darkness and opened a way out one day when I suddenly remembered how much I loved sewing. When I bought my first sewing machine and started sewing as an outlet, I realized just how depressed I really was. Twenty-five years later, I still struggle with depression, though not as severe or lengthy as that time years ago. Now, I am able to identify the emotion more clearly, and I have found ways to emerge from the fog of it sooner rather than later. If anyone tries to tell you depression isn't real, or you're just being "too sensitive" (was accused of that as well), don't listen to the lies.*

We all have days when we feel down, but depression that goes on beyond a few days, or no clear way to get out of it, can become a burden to your soul." – Ana

Signs and symptoms of depression vary among individuals, and usually involve physical, behavioral, and emotional changes. We may conjure up an image of a depressed person lying in bed, crying, and not eating, etc. However, the actual picture may look very different. Sometimes, this individual may not display these outward characteristics. They may participate in a daily routine, go to work, talk and laugh with co-workers and friends, and then return home and sit in front of the television passively waiting for bedtime. Physical signs may include appetite change (eating too much or not enough), skipping meals, sleep disturbances (insomnia or oversleeping), decreased energy, headaches, and unexplained digestive issues. Some of the behavioral changes are loss of interest or lack of passion for activities that were once enjoyed, difficulty concentrating or making decisions, and neglecting responsibilities. The emotional changes that may arise are persistent sadness, crying "for no reason", irritability and anxiety, intrusive thoughts, feelings of hopelessness, loneliness, and sometimes suicidal thoughts. This can affect an individual's ability to perform normal daily activities and may even cause physical pain. Those suffering with depression may experience the impact in a variety of ways—no two individuals will have the exact same symptoms.

A forty-year-old male relative who lost his wife in a car accident over seven years ago expressed his depressive episode like this:

> *"I've been mired in depression for the past two weeks. I don't get out of bed until two o'clock every day. A couple days ago, I slept for twenty-four hours straight. I'm trying to find some way to pull myself out of this, and I just don't know how…—I couldn't get out of bed to bring my children to school. My 14-year-old daughter became the parent. I couldn't do anything… There were times where I just couldn't get out of this cycle of depression, and I just slept because it helped me not to think. If I was sleeping permanently, I wouldn't think or feel anything. "– Greg*

Years after the car accident, Greg shared:

> *"I struggled with alcohol for the last 7 years. I was finally able to get it under control this year and it's been going well. I'm in a much better place than I was, and I've removed negative situations and people from my life. My depression and PTSD has been much better with the help of medications. As we are nearing the anniversary of her death, I'm pretty sure I'll be able to handle it without reverting to my old self."*

Similar to an anxiety disorder, an individual can experience small bouts of depression from time to time. The symptoms of depression can range from mild to severe. For those individuals with major depression, it is common for episodes to last months or years or occur several times throughout their life. Still there are others who may be high-achievers, extroverts, appear confident and happy, and have it all together, and still experience some form of depression. And it's possible for someone with depression to hide their depression from their loved ones, friends, and coworkers. If depression is left untreated, it can lead to substance abuse, abusive behavior, self-harm, and suicide. Suicide is often the final collapse under what appears to be "an unbearable weight".

Therapies

All forms of anxiety and depression can be painful and even serious, especially when you begin to believe that things will never get better, and you feel like nobody understands what you are going through. Depression and anxiety disorders are quite often treated with various types of therapy and medications to manage the disorders in a healthy way. Everyone is different – recommendations for treatment should be based on the individual and the severity of the disorder. There is help available to get people through the difficult times.

Medications

Many individuals with mental health disorders, like depression and generalized anxiety disorder, are steered by medical professionals towards medications such as benzodiazepines and other mor conventional antidepressants (such as Selective Serotonin Reuptake

Inhibitors (SSRIs)) to deal with their mental health disorder. Antidepressants help to manage depression and other mental health disorders by increasing serotonin (a chemical produced naturally in the body) in the brain. Benzodiazepines slow down chemical messages moving between the brain and the rest of the body which help with relaxation of the mind and body. These specific medications are just a few that doctors prescribe to their patients for managing anxiety and depression but there are many others in the marketplace.

Psychotherapies

Psychotherapies are types of counseling that are frequently used for managing moderate depression. This includes Cognitive Behavioral Therapy (CBT) or mindfulness-based cognitive therapy (MCBT). The CBT method is a way of observing your own thoughts and feelings. It attempts to change the way one thinks about certain behaviors and feelings such as fear, failure, loss, rejection, defeat, and helplessness. MCBT is a newer approach that combines cognitive therapy with meditation and promotion of self-kindness based on the creation of mindfulness practice. There are still many other forms of therapy, such as Acceptance Commitment Therapy (ACT) and Eye Movement Desensitization and Reprocessing (EMDR), which are not discussed in this book. A mental health specialist can help you determine which type of treatment is best for you.

Non-Medical Therapies

Treatment for many mental health disorders using nutritional therapy and making lifestyle changes are often not considered by medical doctors as an alternative or complementary way for managing the symptoms associated with these disorders. Throughout this book you will learn about various nutritional and integrative strategies for improving your mental health state such as replenishing your depleted nutrients, reducing refined sugars and processed food, improving your gut bacteria, and exercising. Medical doctors may tell you that "nutrition has nothing to with it." This statement may not be completely accurate. As one researcher noted: "…it would be a pivotal change for psychiatry if specific dietary patterns are definitively demonstrated to prevent or diminish psychiatric disorders in prevalence or severity." Let me be clear, there is no one type of food, specific food plan, exercise program, dietary supplement or combination of foods that can cure depression or anxiety permanently. The use of a combination of nutrition, medication, therapy, or counseling for those with moderate to severe symptoms associated with a mental health disorder may be required. Taking care of your mental health is a lifetime practice and there are sure to be ups and downs. A counselor or therapist will most likely have the skills to help you build your "mental muscle" just like a personal trainer can do with the muscles in your body. However, getting a clear understanding of how nutrition is connected to your mental health can be very helpful with successfully managing anxiety and depression symptoms. As you learn more about the link between food and mental health, you can share the information with your loved ones and friends. Everyone can benefit.

If you are dealing with severe symptoms related to the mental health disorders discussed in this chapter, it is important for you to connect with a licensed healthcare professional who specializes in mental health so you can get the proper diagnosis and treatment. The feelings that may be keeping you from enjoying life are not something you have to live with forever.

CHAPTER TWO

THE GUT-BRAIN CONNECTION

"Every day we live and every meal we eat influence the great microbial organ inside us – for better or worse."

— Giula Enders

Have you ever experienced stomach distress such as abdominal cramps or loose stools during times of heightened anxiety? Did you know that this is probably not a coincidence and that there is a likely explanation for this occurrence? The brain and the gut, also known as the gastrointestinal tract (GI), are connected. A disruption in the gut can send signals to the brain, just as a "troubled" brain can send signals to the gut. Therefore, GI distress can be the cause or the result of anxiety, depression or stress. There is a very complex, bidirectional, and multi-layered relationship between the brain and the gut. It is important to understand that scientists are still conducting lots of new research to understand the connection between the gut and the brain, and how it affects mental health. In this chapter, we will explore this gut-brain connection.

The brain is the main seat of logic and intellect. It is a highly sophisticated and complex organ. It has over 70 billion nerve cells called neurons. Neurons control just about everything we do, and they communicate with each other using chemicals called neurotransmitters by sending "messages" in their own language to each other. There are chemical reactions happening in the brain every second using different types of neurotransmitters– some make neurons more active, and others make them less active. The brain is at work

24/7 to give us the power we need throughout the day, using the "fuel" from the food we eat.

In addition to the brain located in the cranium, scientists now believe that there is a "second brain" located in the gut. This "second brain" contains its own nervous system and manufactures many neurotransmitters. It is also responsible for regulating muscles and hormones, and many other functions, all without any help from the "main brain." The gut is made up of trillions of microbes also known as bacteria. The collection of microbes is called the microbiome. The microbiome is unique with over 1,000 bacterial species; no two people have the same microbiome. These living bacteria residing in your intestine protect the lining of the gut against toxins, help to absorb and digest the nutrients from food, regulate hormones, guide emotions, and activate the messaging pathway between the gut and the brain. Our genes, dietary intake, environment, stress, medications, and other factors help to shape our microbial community. Bacteria within the gut has been shown to influence a vast range of conditions ranging from autism to obesity. The food we eat determines the type of bacteria that will help foster the growth in our gut, which can increase or decrease the risk of several chronic diseases such as anxiety and depression, irritable bowel syndrome (IBS), diabetes, obesity, eczema, and chronic fatigue syndrome. Here is an example of the gut-brain connection as experienced by a female client suffering with many mental and physical ailments:

> *"Two things usually happen when I have anxiety and/or depression. When my anxiety is severe, I feel like ants are crawling throughout my body. I can't sit still, and I tend to eat and drink a lot of comfort foods, like soda and other unhealthy foods, which doesn't help me feel better at all. This type of eating just makes me have bowel movements and/or diarrhea multiple times a day on a regular basis. The same thing happens when my depression becomes severe. However, when my depression is severe and my anxiety is mild, I don't eat very much all day and sometimes I end up hungry late at night. This is when I find myself eating at weird hours which leaves me agitated and restless. Both anxiety and depression mess up my GI." - Sara*

Are you wondering how the brain and gut "talk" to each other? The neurotransmitters that control certain behaviors are produced by the gut and then transported along the pathways that connect nerve cells to the brain. Everything that is produced in the intestines, including the microbiome, will move along this pathway which will affect the functioning of the brain. It can tell us when we are happy, sad, tired or craving something. Eating unhealthy food and using unhealthy substances, such as alcohol, alters the brain's signaling by releasing chemicals from the foods we eat into the gut. This can interfere with the digestion process and can also lead to mood changes or mental health disorders (Figure 2).

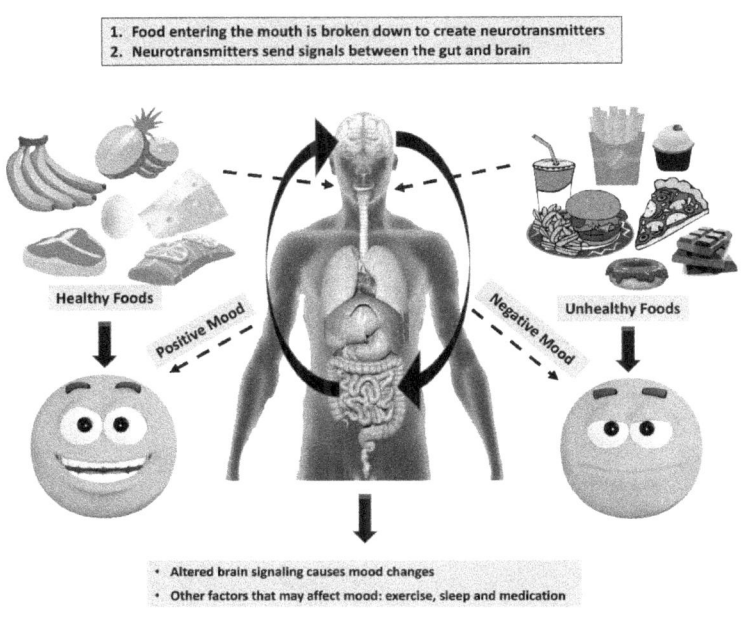

1. Food entering the mouth is broken down to create neurotransmitters
2. Neurotransmitters send signals between the gut and brain

Healthy Foods

Positive Mood

Negative Mood

Unhealthy Foods

• Altered brain signaling causes mood changes
• Other factors that may affect mood: exercise, sleep and medication

Figure 2: Gut Brain Connection

This connection between the gut and the brain dates to ancient times when the digestive system was thought to be the root of our emotions. Today there is evidence that shows feelings of anxiety and stress have a huge impact on the overall sensitivity of the gut, like the "butterflies" you feel when you are anxious or nervous. Dr.

David Perlmutter states in his book, *Brain Maker*, "Although the final straw in triggering an anxiety disorder may very well be misfires in those parts of the brain that control fear and other emotions, we can't negate the fact that such neural transmissions partly depend on the health of the microbiome." The feelings you experience, perhaps sadness, anxiety, happiness or stress can be coming from messages or signals from the gut. It's important to understand this brain-gut connection as it relates to your mental health symptoms. The microbiome can be altered. Any small change to the foods you eat each day can change the bacteria in your gut very quickly. Exploring connections between your "gut" feelings and your "mood" feelings may reveal some needed dietary changes. In a later chapter, I have included valuable information about the various foods you can eat to diversify and encourage the growth of good bacteria.

CHAPTER THREE

THE ROLE OF NUTRITION IN MENTAL HEALTH

"Your body is a temple, but only if you treat it as one."

— Astrid Alauda.

Anthony Bourdain, the television chef who traveled the world indulging in exotic foods and drinks before taking his life, wrote in his memoir: "Your body is not your temple. It's an amusement park." I believe our body is our temple. We often hear common phrases such as: *"You are what you eat"*, *"Tell me what you eat and I will tell you what you are"*, and *"Man is what he eats."* If we really think about it, the food we eat does become part of our body which can then impact our mental health. Have you ever looked at chocolate ice cream in the freezer and thought about how great it tastes and how happy you'll feel eating it? We have all been there. We feel an urge to ease our anxiety, nervousness, or depression by turning to food. But we know that overindulgence can lead to increased body weight and other detrimental effects. What we eat strongly influences our body physically and mentally.

According to the authors of *Understanding Nutrition,* nutrition is defined as "the science of foods and the nutrients and other substances they contain, and of their actions with the body (including ingestion, digestion, absorption, transport, metabolism, and excretion)." Nutrients are substances in our food that our body processes and are required for our bodies to function properly. Human nutrition is broken down into two categories: macronutrients and micronutrients. Macronutrients and micronutrients provide us with the energy we need for our body to move and function. Macronutrients include carbohydrates, protein and amino acids, fats and fatty acids, fiber, and water. Micronutrients include essential vitamins and minerals such as magnesium, selenium, iodine, vitamin B12, and vitamin C. All nutrients are crucial for your health. They are needed to support and promote healthy function of cells, and various processes in our bodies, including the production of neurotransmitters and enzymes.

Nutrition is not only critical for the human body composition, but also has a significant effect on our mental health. One of the newest approaches to help us understand the role nutrition plays in mental health is known as nutritional psychiatry. According to Dr. Uma Naidoo, a Harvard trained nutritional psychiatrist and founder and director of the first hospital-based Nutritional Psychiatry Service in the United States, "What we put on our plate can have powerful outcomes on our physical and mental health, especially as we age." This field of study suggests that the food we consume can affect the severity and risk of common health conditions such as depression, anxiety, schizophrenia, addiction, and other mental health disorders. Thus, dietary changes can be used to treat mental health disorders. Nutritional psychiatrists incorporate foods into their overall treatment plan, and they use nutrition to "optimize brain health and to treat and prevent mental health disorders," according to psychiatrist and author, Drew Ramsey.

Nutritional psychiatry offers a way to connect healthy food with a healthy mind. By eating more foods that are filled with vitamins, minerals, antioxidants, fiber and lean protein and eating less "empty" calorie foods like cookies and cakes, better regulation of various neurotransmitters is achieved. For instance, we know that caffeine stimulates the brain, too much sugar can make children "hyperactive", and chocolate makes us all feel good. And research shows that eating leafy green vegetables such as spinach, kale, and collard greens helps to maintain the function of our neurotransmitters. Nutritional psychiatry is an emerging field that is helping individuals with mental health disorders understand that nutritional factors are interlaced with human emotions.

The relationship between nutrition and mental health starts at a very early stage in life. What our mothers and fathers ate or did not eat, and their consumption of proper nutrients before conception has a significant impact on our mental health. Research shows that maternal and paternal deficiencies in nutrients, such as folate, can increase the risk of anxiety and depressive behaviors in their offspring. The body needs adequate levels of folate to produce neurotransmitters, such as dopamine and serotonin. Unless the body has a good supply of this nutrient, mood problems will result. After a child is born, obtaining good nutritional input continues to be critical, especially for infant brain cognitive development. There is even a link between breast feeding and reduction of mental health disorders. The breast milk from the mother can be a source of beneficial bacteria needed to feed the infant's gut which can reduce the risk of these disorders.

It bears repeating that the determining factors of mental health are complex and there is increasing evidence which indicates a strong link between poor food choices and exacerbation of mental health disorders, including anxiety and depression. It is also known that poor dietary intake leads to nutrient deficiencies or insufficiencies which can change the way the brain functions. Hormonal and blood sugar imbalances, food allergies and sensitivities are also factors that may negatively affect mental health.

Nutrient Deficiencies

"I consider myself a strong woman and therefore able to endure anything, including a pandemic. Then the winter of 2020 arrived, and the weather got cold, the days got shorter, the world introduced a new variant, and we went into lockdown. Within one week, a cloud of anxiety crept in and took over me like a rapid thunderstorm. I couldn't understand what was stirring things up for me. I walked around nervous and feeling discomfort in the pit of my stomach, even when I was simply just watching TV. I spent days battling irrational thoughts around my health, feeling scared about having cancer or another severe illness. It all felt

like a foreign invasion in my body and mind since I had never felt anything like it. I'm cheerful, positive, outgoing, and usually the one who supports and loves on those struggling with life. A friend recommended that I have my vitamin D level checked. My level was low and so I started taking vitamin D supplements daily. After just a couple of days, I noticed the discomfort in the pit of my stomach wasn't taking up as much space."

- Sandy

This is a forty-five-year-old client who eats healthy, exercises daily, has a normal body weight and is experiencing moderate anxiety regularly. Even though she was making healthy lifestyle choices, she was deficient in vitamin D. Many people, like this client, have no idea that they are affected by nutrient deficiencies. One or more vitamin and mineral deficiencies may occur for many reasons and can negatively impact our mental health. Not getting enough nutrients from the foods we eat, and/or not properly absorbing, or digesting them is a significant cause for deficiency. Certain medications, as well as chronic and excessive alcohol consumption, may also be the culprit.

Nutrient deficiency is particularly common with the B vitamins and vitamin D. The B vitamins consist of B1 (thiamin), B2 (riboflavin), B3 (niacin), B5 (pantothenic acid), B6 (pyridoxine), B7 (biotin), B9 (folate), and B12 (cyanocobalamin). B vitamins are involved in many biological processes in the body and are very important for the nervous system, as well as the synthesis of neurotransmitters that regulate our mental function. Because the B vitamins do not get stored in the body, we must get all these vitamins from either the food we eat or dietary supplements. Insufficient and inconsistent intake of these different B vitamins often occurs with unhealthy eating habits, excessive alcohol consumption, and stress.

Vitamin D, the "sunshine vitamin", is responsible for many different functions in the body. But did you know it is also useful in regulating our mental health state? Numerous studies have shown that inadequate levels of vitamin D are linked to higher levels of depression and anxiety. It is important to remember that adequate levels and efficient utilization of vitamin D are needed to make neurotransmitters that regulate our mental function. It is almost impossible to get enough of this vitamin from food. Most food sources, such as salmon, sardines, eggs, and cow's milk, contain only a small amount of vitamin D. Although some foods are fortified with vitamin D, most food sources, such as yogurt, cereals and orange juice, contain only a small amount.

Diet alone does not provide most people with the needed nutrients for optimal health. Fresh vegetables and fruits have lost about 40% of their nutrient value since the 1950s. The nutrient levels have been depleted due to many factors. Food is industrially produced, damaged by heat, exposed to chemicals and pesticides, injected with hormones and antibiotics, and grown in soil that is itself depleted of nutrients. Yet another reason for lower levels of essential nutrients relates to the types of foods we consume in our dietary plan. For instance, individuals consuming the Western diet, also known as the Standard American Diet (SAD), typically eat very few fruits, vegetables, and whole grains. This diet consists mostly of sugar, industrial seed oils (such as canola oil) and ultra-processed foods including hot dogs, fast foods, soda, prepackaged pastries, and breakfast cereals. As a result of the SAD, Americans are deficient primarily in vitamin D, vitamin K, calcium and vitamin C. And finally, there are certain medications (such as high blood pressure medications, acid blockers, antacids, antibiotics) and medical conditions (such as cancer and celiac disease), which can slowly deplete essential minerals and vitamins leading to nutrient deficiencies.

In addition to vitamin and mineral deficiency, inadequate protein intake can also affect mental health. Protein deficiency occurs when your intake cannot meet your body's requirement. Protein is one of the three primary macronutrients that is made up of amino acids which comes directly from the foods we eat. It is an essential nutrient for developing, maintaining, regulating, and repairing almost all the tissues, bones and muscles in our body. Protein provides energy and is needed for proper body function. Amino acids are the building blocks of body tissue and comprise many of the mood regulating neurotransmitters in the brain. One of the main proteins the body uses for creating these neurotransmitters is the amino acid, tryptophan. Pumpkin seeds are a great source of tryptophan as are turkey, chicken, fish, eggs, pineapples, kiwi fruit, plums, plantains, and nuts. The exact amount of protein you need depends on your age, height, body weight and activity level.

Are there ways to tell if you have a nutrient deficiency or if your body is absorbing nutrients properly? One way to determine the level in your blood is through macronutrient and micronutrient analysis testing. Results from these tests, will give you information regarding what you need to eat or drink, and/or lifestyle changes you can make to balance your nutrients. Your healthcare provider can provide a list of specialized labs that can perform these types of tests.

Hormonal Imbalance

When facing mental health issues, like anxiety and depression, it is very easy to overlook the imbalance of hormones. The body needs a balance of stress hormones (such as cortisol and adrenaline), sex hormones (such as estrogen, progesterone, and testosterone) and thyroid hormones (such as T3 and T4) since they are involved in regulating mood and reproductive functions, as well as controlling metabolism. For example, if you experience anxiety, your body will respond by releasing cortisol which can slow digestion and reduce appetite. Hormones help us to keep our body functioning smoothly.

When hormones are out of balance, there will be impact on our food and drink choices, the amount of food we eat, and how often we feel like eating. Poor eating habits (like skipping meals, overeating, or not eating enough), excessive alcohol consumption, inadequate and poor sleep quality, insufficient exercise, and chronic stress are all factors that can disrupt the body's hormone balance and compromise our mental health. This sort of imbalance can cause or worsen existing mental health issues. Many of these changes in food patterns and eating behaviors (such as uncontrolled eating or emotional eating) affect women when hormone levels fluctuate. The hormone levels' fluctuation is very complex. When a woman enters the perimenopause and menopause transition stages of life, which are uniquely challenging periods, she often experiences hormonal changes that may make her more vulnerable to mental health changes.

The sex hormones estrogen, progesterone, and testosterone all play an important role in our mental health. Estrogen and progesterone are mainly produced in the ovaries. These hormones are used to control the woman's reproduction cycles and menstruation, and can influence her mental health state, leading to anxiety, depression, irritability, etc. Testosterone helps in the production of sperm, and can affect the function of the central nervous system. It is important to note that both men and women produce estrogen, progesterone, and testosterone hormones. Women have much higher amounts of estrogen than men, and men have much higher levels of testosterone than women. Hormone fluctuations involving the rise and fall of estrogen happen during menstruation, pregnancy, menopause, and lactation stages in a woman's life. During these times, when there is an increase or decrease in hormones , it is possible to see mental health symptoms increase. When estrogen is low, you may feel anxious and depressed. Low levels of progesterone can result in both anxiety and disturbed sleep. When testosterone levels are low in men, mood, motivation, memory, and strength are affected. Lifestyle changes can improve hormone levels, such as eating healthy food that limits sugar and includes sufficient protein, getting enough exercise, and practicing stress reduction techniques. If you are struggling with your mental health, it is highly recommended that you get your hormone level checked. If you are still menstruating, you should have the test done on day nineteen or twenty of your menstrual cycle.

Blood Sugar Imbalance

Have you ever felt anxious, tired, irritable, or felt a craving for sugar, but felt better after eating something? This could be due to a blood sugar imbalance. When high amounts of refined carbohydrates such as bread, pasta, and pastries are consumed, the glucose level in our blood surges causing a high amount of insulin to be produced. Insulin helps remove the glucose from the blood and move it into our cells. But high levels of insulin lead to a dip in the normal glucose level which then may cause us to feel like we have "crashed". When blood sugar levels dip too low, our adrenal glands produce hormones such as cortisol and adrenaline to help increase the glucose level. The release of adrenaline can result in symptoms of anxiety which can sometimes feel like a panic attack. Cortisol can affect the production of neurotransmitters which then can affect mood. How can you avoid the rapid rise and fall of your blood sugar level? The best way to achieve this is by eating well balanced meals of protein (meat, fish, beans, and legumes), carbohydrates (grains, fruits, and vegetables), and healthy fats (fatty fish, avocados, and nuts).

Food Intolerance

When we think about food intolerance, we might not associate it with mental health. Because some people use the terms "food intolerance" and "food allergy" interchangeably, it is important to understand the difference. A food intolerance occurs when the body cannot digest or break down certain components in food. The most common food intolerances are to gluten (found mainly in wheat, barley, and rye), lactose (found in dairy products), and fructose (found in fruit juices, sweet teas, and soft drinks). Symptoms of a food intolerance may include nausea, bloating, gas, stomach pain, diarrhea, rashes, chronic ear and sinus infections, headaches, or joint pain. A food intolerance reaction may be immediate or delayed. A food allergy typically occurs when your body's immune system responds to a particular food such as cow's milk, nuts, shellfish, soy, and eggs. Food allergies trigger a reaction which can occur anywhere from "a few minutes to two hours after the food is eaten." They cause symptoms that can range in severity from a mild case of hives to difficulty breathing and throat tightness which can be life-threatening.

Food intolerances can affect mental health in several ways. Here is an example of how gluten intolerance can affect mood. Gluten is a protein found in wheat, barley, rye, soy sauce, beer, ice cream, and many packaged foods. An individual with gluten intolerance may sometimes experience inflammation in the gut. The consumption of gluten can result in damage to the intestinal lining of the gut. This damage occurs when undigested protein from gluten enters the blood stream, which then creates further inflammation in other body systems including the brain. Inflammation in the gut makes it difficult to absorb the nutrients needed to create the neurotransmitters that are involved in the regulation of mood. Research shows that chronic inflammation in the gut also affects the brain which can result in symptoms of depression and poor mood regulation. Please note that gluten does not affect all people in this manner. However, for those who are sensitive, gluten can have significant effects on their health.

There are several large studies that have investigated the link between food intolerance and mental health. Based on these studies, scientists believe that food intolerances can cause inflammation and changes to the way neurons react in the brain which leads to depression and anxiety symptoms. If you suspect that food intolerance may be an issue for you and you suffer from depression or anxiety, a food tolerance test and food and symptom journal (see Appendix B) may be able to help you identify particular patterns linking certain foods with mood changes. A healthcare professional or nutritionist can provide information on the food intolerance test that may be right for you.

Poor Eating Pattern

Eating dinner late at night, skipping breakfast or not eating on a regular schedule are also factors that can affect our mental health. Here is how it works.

Every cell in our body has its own internal clock which is regulated by our genes. These clocks control many aspects of your life and they do it continuously. For example, they send signals when it's time to eat and sleep. Our internal clock is a mechanism that keeps track of time within the cell and falls into an approximate 24-hour cycle called the circadian rhythm. The circadian rhythm aligns with your sleep and wake cycle so that you feel more awake in the day and sleepy at night. Even your immune system operates on a 24-hour schedule, guided by the circadian rhythm.

The clocks in the cells stay in rhythm with each other because they are coordinated by a central clock located in the brain, which uses sunlight to synchronize the entire body's circadian rhythm. An irregular circadian rhythm can have profound consequences on your body's physical and mental health. There is evidence that suggest that following a time-restricted eating pattern may improve mood. Time-restricted eating is a form of "fasting" in which an individual only eats between certain hours. This is very different than "traditional fasting" in which someone may abstain from food over the course of a day or longer. Time-restricted eating is typically limited to 10-12 hours. As an example, an individual may limit all food and drink (except water) to the hours between 9:00am and 7:00pm). Various studies found that shift workers, such as night nurses and truck drivers, who ate late at night were less likely to have a regular eating schedule, which then led to increased depression-like and anxiety-like symptoms. When the central clock in your brain is out of sync with your eating pattern, the brain cannot function at full capacity. This means that eating your meals at abnormal times can result in negative mental health outcomes.

As you consider nutrition, don't only think about the content of your food. Also consider the timing of your meals. Do you eat at regular intervals and times? If not, see if you can make changes to establish more regularity. Changing your eating pattern may improve your mental health symptoms. Research supports the benefits of time-restricted eating. It may be just what you need.

CHAPTER FOUR

FOODS AND SUPPLEMENTS TO SUPPORT MENTAL HEALTH

"Let food be thy medicine"

— Hippocrates

Thousands of years ago Hippocrates, the father of modern medicine, authored the famous words, "Let food be thy medicine and medicine be thy food." He knew that various compounds within foods, herbs (e.g., ginseng, gingko biloba, and lemon balm) and spices (e.g., sage and turmeric) contained healing properties, and had the power to nourish, protect and heal our bodies. The foods we eat contain an array of vitamins, minerals and phyto-nutrients to help us achieve healthy digestion, improve mental health, prevent disease, boost metabolism, fight inflammation, and so much more. In essence, food controls almost every function of the body and mind and revitalizes our health. Besides these benefits, food also contains information that tells our genes what to do once within our body. It can change our mood, and in some ways, we become what we feed our mind – whether food or thoughts.

The foods we eat are either beneficial, problematic, or neutral. The beneficial foods tend to be foods that are nutrient-dense. Nutrient-dense refers to foods that are filled with key vitamins, minerals, fiber, antioxidants, and phytonutrients, which are all necessary for the production of neurotransmitters. Dr. Drew Ramsey, nutritional psychiatrist, and Dr. Laura LaChance, nutritional psychiatry researcher, label certain nutrient-dense foods (e.g., goat meat, oysters, butternut squash, spinach, and mustard greens) as "antidepressant foods" since these foods can potentially have antidepression effects. The nutrients in the food we eat allow the body to operate at full capacity. Without it, our body function becomes impaired, and prone to chronic disease. The problematic foods consist of highly processed and packaged foods, as well as sugary foods (e.g., candy, ice cream, cookies, fruit juices, etc.). These foods are often addictive and may worsen anxiety or depression. Providing the body with the right foods will help the brain function at its highest level of performance and as a result our minds become clearer.

Exactly how we absorb, metabolize, and eliminate our food is different for everyone. Some factors that may affect our metabolism include exercise, sleep duration, gut microbiome, and body composition. These factors are often overlooked by nutritionists who make the same food recommendations for each person, using the "one-size-fits all" approach. They fail to recognize that our bodies react differently even though we might eat the same foods. A meal that may be beneficial for one person could be detrimental to another person.

It is important to experiment with different foods to understand what works best for you. Some experts believe that if you have a tendency towards depression, you should eat more grains for breakfast and lunch while consuming very little fat, but lots of protein for dinner. If anxiety is more of a problem for you, then consuming a lot of protein foods for breakfast, such as eggs, meat, veggies, and more starch and fat at dinner time is suggested. Finding the right foods to balance your mental health is not a simple process.

This chapter contains examples of food within categories that are identified as "beneficial" or "problematic". These are just samples—there are many other foods that fall within these categories. As you read through the sections, please don't think of these foods as "good" or "bad." Like David Marc reminds us in his book, *Nourishing Wisdom*, "There is no such thing as an intrinsically good or bad food. Food is neutral. We can assess the effects of food, though, as either desirable or undesirable." Some of these foods you select from the list may make you feel mentally well, while others may not. You can think about it like this. Many medications have various side effects and do not work for some people. Sometimes a process of trial and error is needed to determine what medication works best. The same is true of food. If you want your mental health to improve, try eating a variety of the beneficial foods for an adequate supply of vitamins and minerals, then monitor to see how they make you feel. See if you can find the link between the consumption of certain beneficial foods and improved mental health.

If you consume some of the foods on the problematic list, do so sparingly and pay attention to any adverse effects on your mood. The goal is to reap benefits from the food you eat. Consider keeping a food and mood journal to track what you are eating and drinking and how it makes you feel. I have provided an example of one in Appendix B. Journaling is an effective tool to help you become attuned to the signals your body is sending you.

Beneficial Foods

Research has been conducted on the following foods and has shown they are effective in naturally managing many of the symptoms related to mental health disorders such as anxiety and depression. There is much scientific evidence to support the benefits of these foods which contain super sources of macronutrients, vitamins, minerals, fibers, antioxidants, and beneficial bacteria for creating the neurotransmitters needed to keep you mentally sound. Whatever foods you select from this list, opt for ones that are organic and high-quality when possible. Organic foods have decreased exposure to pesticides, antibiotics, and synthetic fertilizers. High-quality foods are minimally processed, which mean that they will typically contain five or less ingredients and are processed only as much as necessary to enhance or prevent the loss of nutritional value. If buying fish, it should be wild-caught. Try to eat well-balanced meals that contain adequate amounts of carbohydrates, protein, and fats. Stick to foods which are beneficial to the body and avoid those which may trigger anxiety and depression. Many of these foods have personally helped me with my anxiety by naturally increasing various neurotransmitter levels.

Prebiotics and probiotics foods - Prebiotics are carbohydrates that act like a fertilizer to feed or nourish the bacteria in the gut to help them thrive. Probiotics are live bacteria found in fermented foods which are useful for nourishing your gut, balancing neurotransmitters, and protecting the intestinal lining of the gut.

Prebiotics and probiotics are contained in fermented foods and beverages which are produced through a process in which bacteria and yeast break down sugar. Some evidence suggests that individuals with mental health conditions who consume high amounts of fermented food experience a decrease in depressive symptoms. Fermented foods provide nutrients that help to build a healthy and diverse microbiome. The goal is to achieve the right balance – more good bacteria and less bad bacteria. Listed below are examples of prebiotic and probiotic foods:

Prebiotics: Artichokes, bananas, barley, beets, berries, eggplant, flaxseed, garlic, green tea, raw honey, legumes, onions, leeks, peas, rye, shallots, soybeans, wheat

Probiotics: Aged cheese, kefir, kimchi, kombucha, pickles, miso paste, pickled vegetables and fruits, sauerkraut, sourdough bread, tempeh, vinegar, live-cultured yogurt

When purchasing probiotics, be sure to read the label to ensure the product contains live and active culture. Also stay away from products containing excess sugar, which is anything over 5 grams (or 4 teaspoons).

Fruits–All types of berries, apples, bananas, cherries, peaches, grapes, and melons are beneficial for your mental health. Fruits are filled with antioxidants and fiber. Fiber feeds the bacteria in your gut, leading to a healthier and diverse microbiome, which in turns improves mental health. To increase your fiber intake, leave the skin on your fruit—it contains the most fiber. Aim for a variety of fruits.

Here are a few fruits that are particularly helpful for anxiety and depression.

Bananas – Bananas contain over 20% of the recommended daily allowance of vitamin B6. This vitamin can be converted into serotonin, a powerful brain neurotransmitter that is associated with enhancing mood. Perhaps this is one reason why bananas have been shown scientifically to lessen depression and anxiety and improve overall mood. Bananas are also high in potassium, magnesium, and prebiotic fiber. These nutrients are also associated with positive effects on mood, and beneficial for feeding the gut microbiome. Recall that when there are changes to the gut bacteria, there may also be changes to the brain. So, a balanced microbiome in the gut could improve your mental health. From my own experience, eating one banana at the start of the day has helped reduce my anxiety. A banana goes great with nut butter and dark chocolate. It is by far one of my favorite snacks.

Blueberries – Blueberries contain beneficial compounds that can significantly improve depression and reduce both anxiety and stress. These berries can help you beat the blues. Fresh blueberries are great, but frozen blueberries are equally good because they are usually processed and frozen soon after they are picked which minimizes loss of nutrients. Here are some suggestions to incorporate blueberries into your diet: use them as a topping on oatmeal, yogurt, etc.; sprinkle them over green salad; make blueberry sauce by microwaving fresh or frozen berries along with a spoonful of your favorite jelly or jam; add them into your smoothie.

Vegetables – The more vegetables you consume, the better. There is much evidence which indicates that individuals who eat five or more portions (2-3 cups) of vegetables frequently have less stress and mental health symptoms such as depression. Vegetables not only contain high levels of antioxidants, but they also contain fiber to improve the microbiome and mental health. Here are some vegetables that should be included in your regular diet.

Leafy Greens –Kale, spinach, collard greens, turnip greens, and mustard greens are all considered leafy green vegetables. These vegetables receive high priority because they are loaded with nutrients which are crucial to our mental health. Unfortunately, many of us just don't eat enough of these greens. The dislike of vegetables is very common. A male client once shared that when he was six years old his mother told him that he could not leave the table until the vegetables disappeared—He stuffed them up his nose. Don't care to eat leafy greens in a salad? Try adding them to a smoothie, sauté in olive oil or mix into soups. You can't go wrong with these nutrient-dense greens.

Mushrooms – Edible mushrooms are a group of foods that can be significantly beneficial to mental health disorders such as anxiety and depression. They contain the highest dietary source of the amino acid called ergothioneine, which is an antioxidant that may protect against cell and tissue damage in the body. Several studies have shown that antioxidants contained in mushrooms can help alleviate mental health disorders such as depression, anxiety, and bipolar disorder. The reishi mushroom has potent medicinal properties and is like nature's anti-anxiety medication. What makes this type of mushroom unique is its ability to calm due to the mood-boosting compound, triterpene. The good news is that you don't have to eat a lot to reap the benefits. There are various types of fresh edible mushrooms that can be added to your diet besides reishi. Lion's mane, cordyceps, enoki, shiitake, maitake, portabella, crimini are all good choices. Most of these varieties can be found in the produce aisle of a natural food store. Mushrooms are sold in a variety of forms, including tea, hot cocoa, coffee, capsules, powder, tinctures, and energy bars. If you buy them fresh, try slicing them and sauteing in a little olive oil. Maybe you'd prefer adding them to a pizza or salad. No matter how you decide to consume mushrooms, they are a great way to naturally support your mental health.

Dark chocolate/Cacao – This decadent-sweet treat contains a phytoestrogen ("phyto" means plant) that naturally occurs in plants. Phytoestrogens can increase the levels of neurotransmitters. Chocolate also contains an amino acid called tyrosine, which is linked to an increase in dopamine. Dopamine and endorphins get released during moments of emotional euphoria and have much the same effect on the brain as the active ingredient in marijuana, THC, helping you feel less anxious and more relaxed. According to researchers, healthy adults who consumed dark chocolate containing 85% cacao could significantly alter the diversity of the gut bacteria and improve their mood. It is best to consume dark chocolate that contains at least 70% cacao. Also, remember that chocolate contains caffeine which can contribute to anxious feelings for some people, but may be helpful for those who experience depressive symptoms.

Nuts and Seeds – These plant-based foods are high in protein, fiber, and healthy fat (omega-3). Most nuts contain an amino acid called tryptophan which our body uses to make serotonin to support our mood and reduce stress. Pumpkin seeds, walnuts, cashews and sunflower seeds are all good sources. Consider walnuts. Walnuts have multiple active compounds that can stimulate the production of neurotransmitters such as serotonin that helps us feel more relaxed and calm. Research suggests that people who eat walnuts may decrease depression symptoms compared to those who do not eat any kind of nuts. Cashews are also beneficial for anxiety and depression because they contain magnesium which has positive effects on the nervous system.

Herbs and Spices – For centuries before the invention of pharmaceutical drugs, different cultures all over the world have used herbs and spices for medicinal purposes. Did you know that many drugs have been derived directly from herbs and spices? You can support your mental health by adding culinary herbs and spices to your meals. Not only are they packed with lots of powerful nutrients, but they add flavor as well.

Turmeric is an example of a spice that is beneficial for reducing anxiety and elevating mood. It has hundreds of active compounds that are all beneficial to our health. The mild and distinctive taste of turmeric makes it a common ingredient in many curry dishes. It not only has antioxidant and anti-inflammatory properties, but it can change the activities of our genes that are associated with our mood. Research has shown that it is also beneficial in treating depression symptoms. Turmeric can be consumed as a seasoning/ spice or as a dietary supplement. One down-side to turmeric is that the body is not very good at absorbing it. But one way that you can harness the power of this spice is by combining it with black pepper and coconut oil to help your body absorb it more easily.

Beverages

Green tea – Green tea is rich in compounds such as L-theanine which have an anti-anxiety effect and is calming for the nervous system. A warm cup of tea can be very relaxing. However, getting the medicinal benefit of green tea requires you drink at least six cups daily. This is probably a bit unrealistic for many of us. Instead, you may want to consider a L-theanine supplement which will be described later in this chapter. Do note that some green tea is high in caffeine, so it is best to drink it early in the day. If caffeine gives you the jitters, then drink decaf green tea instead. Some decaffeinated tea has the same health benefits.

Caffeine-free drinks – This category includes all types of herbal tea (e.g., chamomile, peppermint, and hibiscus), and unsweetened plant-based milk (e.g., almond, cashew, oat, coconut, rice, hemp, and soy). A word of caution – drinking too much hibiscus tea can have a laxative effect. Herbal teas contain many active compounds that are useful for increasing neurotransmitter activity, resulting in positive effects on anxiety. Plant-based milks are beneficial since they are fortified with vitamin D, which can increase serotonin levels.

Water – The body is made up mostly of water. Our brain functions properly only when we consume adequate amounts. Without adequate intake of water, the brain will not perform optimally. I cannot emphasize enough the importance of getting plenty of water. With proper hydration, you will think and feel better. Dehydration can occur if we experience anxiety. When we are anxious, sweating increases, which in turn leads to water loss. You can consume different types of water to quench thirst. Just pick your favorite. Choices include tap water, filtered water, spring/glacier water, mineral water, purified water, coconut water, alkaline water and well water. Whatever kind of water you choose, start your morning with a full glass, set specific targets for water intake throughout the day, and carry a bottle with you wherever you go. If you find it difficult to drink plain water because it's tasteless, add a bit of lemon, strawberry, watermelon, or cucumber to it. You can also utilize powdered electrolyte drink mixes with no added sugars or artificial sweeteners.

Problematic Foods

Sugar – This may be the single worst food substance that can negatively impact our mental health. Research shows that over time the consumption of foods with added sugars is linked to depression. When we eat large amounts of sugar, our body reacts by producing large doses of insulin (a hormone that helps to remove excess sugar from the blood) which then provides a quick energy boost. But as soon as the blood sugar level peaks, it quickly drops causing a "sugar crash" which worsens symptoms of anxiety. Many of the foods we eat contain processed sugar which is often referred to using terms such as "artificial sweeteners", "non-sugar sweeteners" and "low-calorie sweeteners." Artificial sweeteners, such as high fructose corn syrup, aspartame, sucralose, and saccharin, are usually not healthy alternatives to sugar and are 200 times sweeter than natural sugar. They have no nutrients and enter the bloodstream very quickly which causes spikes in blood sugar levels. This is not the case for the natural sugars found in fruits and some fruit juices. Additionally, a recent study in 2022, demonstrated common artificial sweeteners change the gut microbiome in humans. Although the mechanism that connects changes in gut microbiome to consumption of artificial sweeteners is unknown, researchers know that these sweeteners change the intestinal bacteria. When bacteria in the gut is modified, there can be detrimental impact to the movement of glucose from the blood into muscle and fat, which can lead to weight gain and diabetes. Make the effort to reduce sugar intake. An easy way to get started is by paying close attention to the "added sugar" contained in many foods, and reading the ingredients on food labels. Look for words like "syrup", "nectar", "molasses", "honey", "corn sweetener", "cane juice", "fruit juice", "barley malt", "sucrose", "fructose", and "dextrose." So, think twice before you reach for that pastry or soft drink.

Caffeine – What's the first thing you associate with caffeine? Are you imagining the smell of a freshly brewed pot of coffee? According to National Coffee Association (NCA), coffee is the most widely consumed beverage in America. There are individuals who can drink up to 4 cups or more of coffee daily and feel energized. However, coffee is only one of the main sources of caffeine and should be considered more like a drug than a beverage. Caffeine is a naturally occurring stimulant found in over 60 plant species and is naturally contained in coffee, tea (green, black, white, matcha), and cocoa. It is added to many products including soda, energy drinks, and some over-the-counter medication. Caffeine's effect on the body depends on how your body metabolizes, absorbs, and utilizes caffeine, how much caffeine you consume, your lifestyle (e.g., sleep and stress), and your physical activity. Some of us are "slow" metabolizers of caffeine while others are "fast" metabolizers. A slow metabolizer will process caffeine at a slower rate, resulting in a more stimulating effect. A fast metabolizer will process caffeine at a faster rate with no lasting effect. When consumed in small amounts, it is fine. At higher quantities caffeine can trigger or exacerbate anxious feelings, particularly for people with anxiety disorders. An excessive amount of caffeine stimulates the nervous system, which can trigger stress hormones that raise your heart rate and release sugar into the blood stream, resulting in heart palpitations, insomnia, and even panic attacks. It is best to experiment to find the right amount of caffeine you can tolerate without adverse effects on your health. Look for caffeine-free options for your favorite beverages. This client's story summarizes the stimulating effects caffeine had on her.

"Sometime last year, I was waking up during the night with occasional chest pain (slight and short) in my left breast area. One night I could not go back to sleep and the pain seemed worse than it's been the other nights. I thought of calling 911 as I was thinking it might be stress related and it could also be a heart attack, but I convinced myself that it was nothing. However, I called my doctor in the morning and told him about the fluttering and palpitations, and anxious feelings I was experiencing. I got an appointment immediately and he performed an ECG/ EKG. The results from this test were negative for heart issues. He asked how much food I ate before going to bed and how much coffee I drank during the day. "I don't drink coffee", I

said. He shared with me that too much caffeine can cause these feelings. But what I did not tell him was that I drink regular black tea. Sometimes I used to drink several cups of black tea (especially during the pandemic lockdown) and I usually left the tea bag in the cup for a long time which would make it extra strong. As it turned out I was overdosing on caffeine from the black tea. I now drink herbal tea instead of black tea. I am sleeping through the night, less anxious and feeling better overall. However, on occasion, I will have a cup of black tea, but I limit it to one cup early in the day. I sometimes have other foods containing caffeine, like a piece of chocolate cake, but it does not affect me as much as the black tea. "- Valerie

As a side note, energy drinks not only contain caffeine, but they are also packed with other ingredients which can be harmful. These drinks are loaded with sugar (one energy drink can have more than 50 grams of added sugar), artificial sweeteners and other additives. Consuming energy drinks can rob the body of important nutrients and disrupt the gut bacteria which can leave you feeling depressed. Energy drinks may temporarily boost your energy, but there is mounting evidence that they can exacerbate symptoms of anxiety and depression. If you want to energize yourself and improve your mood, try going for a brisk walk or taking a power nap.

Alcohol – This is one of the most common substances people use to manage their mental health. Alcohol may be the culprit for significant mood swings and worsening anxiety. For individuals with depression and anxiety, excessive alcohol consumption leads to a vicious cycle. Once consumed, alcohol can temporarily act as both an anti-anxiety and antidepressant agent, but once this effect wears off, it can lead to worsening symptoms of your mental health disorder. For example, having two glasses of alcohol every night after work will probably make you feel relaxed in the short term. But once the feeling wears off, your body goes into withdrawal, and before you know it, you've become more depressed, anxious, or angry. Regular alcohol consumption at any level will most likely have negative effects on your mental health. As such, you should exercise caution around its use. The U.S. Department of Health and Human Services, recommends no more than one drink per day for women, and a limit of two drinks per day for men.

Processed Foods – Highly processed food dramatically influences the entire body, which includes your mental health. Cookies, crackers, chips, and fried foods are all examples of highly processed foods. For example, the white flour in cookies will quickly be converted to glucose in the blood as soon as you eat it. That can cause a rapid spike and then drop in blood sugar which tends to worsen anxiety. Highly processed foods lack fiber, are low in micronutrients, and contain dyes and artificial sweeteners. They also contain additives and preservatives such as MSG. Excessive consumption of these foods are all linked to anxiety and depression problems.

Dietary Supplements

Dietary supplements serve an important role in combating nutrient deficiencies and at the same time they can manage many mental health symptoms. It is a myth that there is not sufficient scientific evidence to support their use. In fact, many supplements are backed by more scientific literature than some of the medications and vaccines that we take.

Several well-researched nutrients that are important for addressing mental health disorders include the following: B vitamins (B6, B9, B12), vitamin D, omega-3, magnesium, zinc, selenium, chromium, and iron. Probiotics, herbals (e.g., ashwagandha, rhodiola, passionflower), and antioxidants (e.g., curcumin and resveratrol) are also helpful in dealing with mental health symptoms. Antioxidants are compounds found in many colorful plant foods which protect the body against free radicals or unstable molecules that increase the risk of various diseases. These plants act like "chill pills" that are great for squashing anxiety and depression.

Although it's always best to get nutrients from whole foods (or foods in their natural form, minimally processed, and without preservatives, added sugars, and other additives), it's becoming increasingly harder to meet all our needs this way. With smart supplementation containing the right nutrients, we can help bridge the gap. What you eat dictates what nutrients you may need to supplement. For example, vegans and vegetarians are at risk of deficiencies in essential nutrients, especially if they are not getting enough vitamin B12. In this case, B12 supplements can assure adequate daily intake.

Appendix A provides a guide for choosing quality supplements. Before you decide to take any of the supplements on this list, it is important to talk with your healthcare provider, especially if you are pregnant, breast feeding or taking medications.

L-theanine

L-theanine is an amino acid that naturally occurs in green, black, and white tea leaves, and some types of mushrooms. One of the great benefits of L-theanine is its ability to naturally reduce stress and anxiety. It does this by boosting levels of neurotransmitters, such as dopamine. A recent study stated that L-theanine "has the potential to promote mental health in the general population with stress-related ailments and cognitive impairment." Here is the catch – someone would have to drink at least six cups of tea every day before they would start to feel improvement in their anxiety. For this reason, a supplement would be far more convenient. I was first introduced to this supplement by my naturopathic doctor following my second anxiety attack. This client with a similar anxiety issue shares her experience about the soothing properties of this supplement:

> *'I have used the amino acid, l-theanine supplement for several years to counteract stress and anxiety without the side effect of drowsiness. I take it in capsule form on a daily basis, as well as by drinking tea (green, black, or white teas) or eating legumes. Whenever I have stopped using l-theanine for a few days, my anxiety increases, so my body needs this supplement." - Nancy*

Omega-3

Omega-3 are types of polyunsaturated fatty acids (PUFAs): eicosapentaenoic acid (EPA), docosahexaenoic acid (DHA) and alpha-linolenic acid (ALA). These types of omega-3 are sometimes referred to as omega-3 fatty acids. PUFAs play a role in regulating immunity and inflammation, mood regulation, energy production and many other processes within the body. DHA and EPA are found mainly in fish or fish oil. ALA is contained in many plants, nuts, seeds, flax seed oil, and some green vegetables. PUFAs are not produced by the body which means we must get them from the foods we eat or from dietary supplements.

For decades, numerous studies investigated the use of omega-3 fatty acids in the management and prevention of depression and other mental health disorders. One study found that medical students with anxiety symptoms who took omega-3 supplements showed a 20% reduction in anxiety. Another study found that menopausal women who took a fish oil supplement had decreased depression symptoms. If you are considering a daily omega-3 supplementation, be sure to choose a high-quality and mercury-free fish oil, algae oil, flax seed, or krill oil supplement containing at least 1000 mg of EPA and DHA. For individuals who don't like fish, or who are vegetarians and vegans, algae sources (e.g., seaweed, spirulina, chlorella, kelp, nori, kombu) are good options for obtaining sufficient EPA and DHA.

Fish oil supplements are available in liquid, capsule and pill form and are generally safe when used as recommended.

Magnesium

Magnesium is one of the most important minerals in your body. It is involved in over 300 functions and reactions related to your heart, nervous system, hormones, and blood sugar. When your magnesium level is low, stress takes over, anxious thoughts persist, and muscles tighten making it very hard to relax. According to a recent 2019 analysis, it was found that "lower serum magnesium levels are associated with depressive symptoms," and researchers recommended the use of magnesium supplementation for the treatment of depression. Other studies show that magnesium supplementation may be helpful in the treatment of mild anxiety and stress-related symptoms.

Magnesium depletion or deficiency can occur for various reasons such as being on a Standard American Diet (SAD), using certain medications (e.g., high blood pressure medications, gastroesophageal reflux disease (GERD) medications), and having various medical conditions. Signs of magnesium depletion may include headaches, muscle cramping, higher blood pressure and anxiety. The following foods are good sources of magnesium: bananas, avocados, broccoli, spinach, dark leafy greens, almonds, cashews, flax seeds, pumpkin seeds and chia seeds, walnuts, beans, chickpeas and peas, dark chocolate, and fatty fish.

If you aren't getting sufficient magnesium from these foods, a supplement may be beneficial. There are various forms of magnesium supplements: glycinate, acetyl taurate, oxide, and citrate. Each supplement can be consumed as a pill, liquid, or oil. Not everyone can tolerate magnesium supplements because of a possible gastrointestinal (GI) side effect. For those dealing with anxiety and depression, magnesium glycinate is a good choice. However, it should be noted that magnesium supplements can interact with medications. So, as with all other supplements, it is important that you, along with your healthcare provider, look at your complete medication and supplement list to review possible interactions.

Vitamin D

It is essential for our bodies to have adequate levels of vitamin D. This vitamin helps to regulate the central nervous system, which can sometimes be dysfunctional in individuals suffering from anxiety and depression. Most of the vitamin D we get is from exposure to the sun. It is the only vitamin that is produced independently by the body through sun exposure, and this exposure is absolutely the best source of vitamin D. It is also important to know that vitamin D requires the presence of other nutrients, such as magnesium, to be adequately absorbed and activated in the body.

The amount of sun exposure you need to create enough vitamin D will depend on many factors, including the amount of sunlight exposure you get without a sunscreen (sunscreen with SPF factor of 8 or greater reduces production of vitamin D by 95%), skin color or tone, genetics, diet, overall health, season of year, location, and air pollution. Skin color is an extremely important factor. People with dark-skin pigments have a greater chance of vitamin D deficiency due to a higher level of melanin which acts as natural sun protection. Research shows that dark-skinned people require 6 times more sun exposure to produce the equivalent amount of vitamin D as light-skinned people.

Although the body is good at creating and storing vitamin D from the UVB light that lands on our skin, this may not be enough to give your body the immediate boost it needs. In this case, taking a vitamin D supplement is suggested. Don't think that because you live in Florida, California, Arizona, or other sunny locations this does not apply to you. Many people spend most of their time indoors. Others may be taking medications that necessitates avoidance of the sun. Also, if you are driving in your car or sitting by a window, assuming you get the sunshine you need, it is important to know that glass blocks UVB ultraviolet light—only minimal vitamin D can be accessed by sun rays in this manner.

At this point, you might be wondering how to know what your vitamin D level is. The level can be determined by a simple blood test. Since vitamin D levels vary depending on the season of the year, make sure you get tested in the middle of the winter and then again in the summer. The reference range for adequate vitamin D varies on the laboratory performing the test. However, as a functional nutritionist, I recommend that my clients aim for a range between 60 and 80 ng/mL. If you decide to take a supplement, I strongly suggest taking a high-quality vitamin D3 supplement (capsule, pill, or liquid) because this form is most like that which is naturally produced in the human body via sunlight exposure. It is also a good idea to take a vitamin D3 supplement with high fat foods such as avocado, salmon, and olive oil to enhance the absorption of vitamin D into the bloodstream.

Ashwagandha

Ashwagandha, also known as "Indian ginseng", is an important and powerful herb that has been used for thousands of years in Ayurvedic medicine to help protect the central nervous system. Ayurvedic medicine is a medical system that uses natural approaches to diagnose and treat various medical conditions. It is believed that ashwagandha can reduce stress and promote relaxation. It can also work as a strong anti-anxiety and antidepression medicine. Ashwagandha has been studied extensively for years. The European Scientific Journal states that "Depression is a pervasive and impairing illness affecting women twice more than men. An ayurvedic approach of using herbs like Ashwagandha seems to be more acceptable to relieve anxiety, stress, depression...". Ashwagandha supplements are made from the root of the plant, and they come in various forms, including capsules, raw powder, and liquid. It's important to remember you will need to take it regularly to reap the long-term benefits.

B-Complex

B-Complex vitamins are greatly underutilized in the management of anxiety and other mental health disorders. Among the B-complex vitamins which are most effective for managing anxiety and depression are vitamin B12 (cobalamin), vitamin B9 (folate), and vitamin B6. Low levels of the B-complex vitamins have been associated with the risk of developing depressive symptoms.

Vitamin B12 is well known as the "energy vitamin" and has an impressive list of functions: maintaining red blood cell formation, promoting immune system function, producing neurotransmitters, maintaining a healthy brain, and managing nervous system functions. A lack of this vitamin can cause serious problems affecting our mental health. There are many factors that can negatively impact B12 levels, such as medications (e.g., antacids and acid blockers), as well as gastric and autoimmune conditions. When your body cannot absorb B12 into the gastrointestinal tract, it becomes depleted of this vitamin. Vitamin B12 is primarily found in animal-source foods, such as fish, meat, poultry, eggs, and dairy products. For many of us, vitamin B12 can be obtained from our diet. But, for others who are following a strict vegetarian or vegan diet, supplementing with B12 may be necessary, especially if testing indicates a depletion of this vitamin.

The other B-complex vitamin needed for healthy mental health is vitamin B9 also known as folate. Folate helps synthesize DNA, repair DNA, and prevent anemia. Folate deficiency may lead to anxiety and depression. Some studies claim that folate may reduce depression when combined with vitamin B12. Various factors that increase risk of folate deficiency are poor-quality diet, alcoholism, genetics, medications, and autoimmune conditions. Folate is found in a variety of foods and is added to some foods, like cereals, in the form of synthetic folic acid.

Other Supplements

Other supplements that may offer some help when dealing with anxiety and depression disorders include GABA and vitamin C. GABA, also known as Gamma-aminobutyric acid, is a neurotransmitter that helps to regulate the nervous system activity. GABA has shown promote relaxation by increasing calming, focused brain waves, while reducing other brain waves associated with worry. Vitamin C may also be helpful since adequate levels of this vitamin are needed for the conversion of the neurotransmitters that are important in the management of depression and mood swings. According to some researchers, vitamin C may even increase the effectiveness of antidepressants.

Final Remarks

Supplements can be a useful complement to other anxiety and depression reducing therapies. Supplements alone won't help you if you are not consuming beneficial foods, and getting regular physical exercise, sufficient sleep, and sunlight. It's very easy to fall into the trap of taking supplements to compensate for poor diet and lifestyle habits. However, taking dietary supplements should not be used as some kind of "quick fix" so you can keep going. It's worth taking the time to determine if you need the support of supplements.

CHAPTER FIVE

THERAPIES FOR BETTER MENTAL HEALTH

*"Choices are at the root of every one of your results. Each choice
starts a behavior that over time becomes a habit"*

— Darren Hardy

We are what we eat, but when it comes to managing mental health such as anxiety and depression, food alone isn't the answer. When we combine medical treatment, diet, and supplements with other therapies such as exercise, arts and crafts, and music, we have the power to improve symptoms of anxiety and depression. It's crucial to have activities that divert our attention away from things that may be arousing our nervous system or making us feel overly anxious or depressed. The goal of these therapies is to help you experience better mental health. Although continuing to learn throughout life is important, enjoying life is important too. Having fun is a crucial step we can take to improve our mental state.

This chapter contains a list of suggested therapies you can try using to help distance yourself mentally from the source of your anxiety and/or depression. These therapies all can have a positive impact on mental health. I encourage you to find one that makes you feel good, involves having fun, and is something you will sustain over a long period of time. If you try a specific therapy and it doesn't work for you, try another one. Remember that it takes time and practice to obtain positive results and see improvements.

Cooking

For years, experts have been encouraging people who are struggling with poor mental health to start cooking or baking. "Culinary therapy" is a trending treatment used by numerous mental health clinics and therapists as a way for patients with mental health disorders to maintain their daily living and distract them from problems. In a 2004 study published in the British Journal of Occupational Therapy, researchers found that baking classes increased concentration, and provided a sense of achievement for patients being treated in an inpatient mental health facility. Cooking is an act of mindfulness, a creative outlet, and a method of communication which is great therapy for soothing stress, increasing self-confidence, and curbing negative thinking. Ultimately, cooking therapy can nourish and calm the mind.

Cooking can take hours or minutes. No matter how much time you spend, cooking can improve anxiety and depression because you need to keep focus on the task at hand – prepping, stirring, mixing—all of which are activities which keep your mind off things that may be making you feel anxious or perhaps depressed. Think of it like meditation with a tasty outcome, like blueberry muffins or herb roasted chicken. How rewarding is that – to eat something that you made yourself, while improving your mental health at the same time? If you choose cooking as your therapy of choice and you feel like you need a little help getting started, you may want to try scrolling through recipes online or buy cookbooks to find healthy, simple, and quick ones that you can tackle, using ingredients you might already have in your kitchen. It is important to remember that you don't have to become a chef.

Gardening

My dad was the best vegetable gardener that I have ever known. He was able to grow delicious tomatoes, Jamaican callaloo (similar to spinach), okra, onions, peppers, beans, and zucchini despite his garden being in the dry and hot desert region. Gardening was his favorite form of relaxation, and it was where he found peace and contentment. It was a way to keep his hands and mind busy. I never thought about it much before, but realize now that when you are digging, planting, weeding, and trimming, you are replacing those anxious and negative thoughts with positive ones. There is new research to support this idea that gardening activities can lower anxiety and depression. Researchers found that healthy women who participated in biweekly gardening sessions were able to reap mental health benefits. Gardening may be your happy place. You can only know if you give it a try.

Hobbies

Finding time to engage in an activity you enjoy is an excellent non-medical intervention that can be an addition to other treatments for depression, anxiety, or stress. Research shows that having a hobby is associated with lower levels of depression and might even prevent depression for some people. If you begin losing interest in things you normally like doing, also known as anhedonia, finding a hobby may be just what you need. Psychologists sometimes treat patients with mild to moderate depression with this type of intervention to relieve their symptoms and bring them pleasure. They believe that participating in an enjoyable hobby can release dopamine which can make us more motivated to continue the activity.

Try hobbies that might ignite a new passion or provide a creative outlet like photography, fishing, pottery or sewing. Puzzles and word games may also be good choices as a way of soothing emotions such as nervousness and sadness. Sometimes taking a class can spark an interest in a specific hobby. You might also want to consider drawing, painting, or coloring which do not require much artistic skill or expensive tools. Some people see a positive effect within just minutes of drawing. Drawing is a powerful way, for me personally, to decrease my anxiety and elevate my mood. The thought of creating something new brings me excitement.

Music/Calming Sounds

"Music makes more people milder and gentler, more moral and more reasonable" – Martin Luther, Theologian

Martin Luther was right; music can make you feel gentler. Have you ever just felt better after listening to your favorite song? As it turns out, listening to music may reduce anxiety and depression by relieving mental anguish. Some experts have noted that calming music can induce a peaceful state. Music therapy can help people feel less anxious especially when facing stressful situations such as surgery.

Listening to calming music is helpful for anxiety while upbeat music seems to be very beneficial for depression. So next time you need a little mood boosting, listen to your favorite music, and start singing and dancing.

But it's not only listening to music that can help you feel better, listening to white-noise and nature sounds can also increase serotonin. White noise is a type of noise that is produced when sounds from all different frequencies are combined. You can access white noise and nature sounds on YouTube or purchase a white noise machine.

Writing/Journaling

Another great way to enhance or boost your mental well-being is by writing or journaling. Writing has been shown to reduce symptoms of anxiety, depression, and physical stress, while enhancing cognitive functioning. To begin writing, find a quiet and comfortable place where you can let your words flow freely. You can document anything and everything—what you are doing, who you are with, thoughts you have, and how you feel. It may seem daunting to write all this down but once you get started, you may become more motivated as you begin to see improvements in your mental and psychological health. In addition to writing down your thoughts, I suggest writing down what you are grateful for each day. Researchers found that people who express more gratitude have lower levels of depression. Gratitude journaling is a good way of shifting negative feelings towards positive ones. I keep a journal right by my bed, so I remember to express and record my gratitude daily.

Physical Exercises

Physical activity is often overlooked as a form of treatment to address depression and anxiety. But exercise and movement can have a powerful healing effect. It is understandable that when feeling poorly, the idea of exercise is not very appealing. Some people equate exercise with long hours at the gym and shun the idea. But exercise doesn't have to involve rigorous workouts. Doing some form of movement like running, jumping rope, dancing, hiking, or walking, are all things that can engage your body and uplift your mood. There are a myriad of exercises you can try. Here are some suggestions to get your heart pumping: brisk walking, jogging, running, playing tennis, swimming, and bicycling. But there are other types of exercises such as yoga, tai chi, and qigong that are also beneficial in reducing anxiety and promoting relaxation. It is important that whatever exercise you choose, make sure it is one that you will enjoy and do regularly. When using physical exercise for managing depression or anxiety, start slowly, if necessary, with five-minute sessions and slowly build up to 20 to 30 minutes daily, seven days a week. The bottom line is that we need a healthy mind to achieve a healthy body, and both require equal attention. Remember taking care of your health, means taking care of your mind and body.

Mental Exercises

Anxiety and panic attacks are terrifying experiences. It is very easy to let the anxious thoughts and feelings take you over. However, you can perform mental exercises which can help you manage these episodes. Here are a few you might try:

Guided Imagery – With this technique you imagine yourself in a happy and comfortable place, perhaps the beach. As you picture yourself in this place, use all your senses to notice all the details. Ask yourself "what do I smell, hear, feel with my hands and feet?"

5-4-3-2-1 Coping Technique – This technique uses the five senses to redirect your mind to concentrate on things in your environment and refocus your attention. Identify 5 things that you can see, 4 things you can touch, 3 things you can hear, 2 things you can smell, and 1 thing you can taste.

Count Down – This technique requires counting backwards from 100 in multiples of 7, which can allow you to focus on the counting and not your anxious thoughts.

Breathing

Did you realize that the way you breathe can impact your mental health? Taking deep breaths regulates your heart rate, opens your blood vessels and carries more oxygen to the brain. Breathing exercises have been shown to help with relaxation and overall mood. According to James Nestor, author of *Breath: The New Science of a Lost Art*, learning to breathe properly can help tame anxiety, depression, PTSD, and other disorders. He suggests that when you inhale and exhale through your nose, your whole body relaxes. Breathing exercises should be done for a few minutes each day to form a habit. Then you will have a useful tool that is always available during times of stress and tension. It should be noted that these techniques don't work for everyone and for some, they can increase a feeling of anxiety. They also may not be appropriate when suffering from fatigue. Below is a list of some breathing exercises you can try. Nestor's book contains additional ones as well.

4-7-8 Breathing or Relaxing Breath – Find a comfortable seat and sit with shoulders back and your back completely straight. Rest the tip of your tongue on the roof of your mouth behind the back of your teeth. Take a few breaths before getting started. Inhale through the nose with lips closed and count to four. Hold your breath for a count of seven and exhale through the mouth for a count of eight. Repeat four more times, and then let your breath return to its own natural rhythm.

Box Breathing – Just like with the 4-7-8 breathing technique, find a comfortable seated position with shoulders back and your back completely straight. Inhale for four counts, hold for four counts, exhale for four counts and rest for four counts.

Respiratory Sinus Arrythmia – This process requires you to take a double inhale through your nose and a long-extended exhale through the nose.

Meditation

There is much research that proves that meditation is very beneficial to your mental health. Meditation found its way into Western therapeutic practices sometime in the twentieth century to reduce anxiety, depression, and stress. Meditation is like an exercise which can be used to reset and clear your mind. You can think of it as a tool intended to help develop mindfulness (focusing solely on the present moment), self-awareness, and focused attention — all of which support mental health. It has been practiced in various cultures all over the world for thousands of years, and nearly every religion uses some form of meditation practice. However, many people practice meditation independently of religion. There are multiple ways to meditate and many different types of meditation. One type of meditation is called mindfulness meditation in which you sit quietly while focusing on your breathing to direct attention away from negative feelings. Some research suggests that this mindfulness meditation may be as effective as Cognitive-Behavioral Therapy (CBT) at easing depression and anxiety symptoms. Guided meditation sessions are also very helpful. These sessions, which are available through apps such as Selfpause, Headspace, and Calm have helped me learn to sit calmly and repeat empowering truths and affirmations. Meditation has become a regular part of my daily routine in the long-term management of my anxiety. You can look for more information on meditation through classes in your local community, YouTube videos and books.

Prayer

Whether you are a believer in God or not, there is much research showing that prayer for healing is often requested and appreciated when people are facing a major illness. There is some evidence to support better outcomes from various medical conditions for those who practice prayer. Furthermore, researchers note that prayer can also be an effective tool in reducing depression and anxiety. Prayer should not be likened to requesting wishes be granted by a genie. Then what exactly is prayer? According to Billy Graham, the renowned evangelist and preacher, "Prayer is spiritual communication between man and God, a two-way relationship in which man should not only talk to God but also listen to Him." Prayer can help make you feel relaxed and can be used as a tool to release stressors of life. I use the Bible to guide me in my prayers. A favorite passage is found in Philippians 4:6-7 which says: "Be anxious for nothing, but in everything by prayer and supplication with thanksgiving let your requests be made known to God. And the peace of God, which surpasses all comprehension, will guard your hearts and your minds in Christ Jesus." Verses like these are a comfort to me. I want to stress that although I believe in the power of prayer, I am not suggesting its use in lieu of medical treatment, but rather to accompany it along with other beneficial non-medical therapies.

Nature

> *"Months ago, I interviewed for a new management position at my job and was rejected for this position. I had been working hard towards this goal for years. This put me in a state of depression for weeks afterwards. `And I figured I needed some type of therapeutic outlet that didn't include a bottle of wine. I chose the great outdoors. I started to take more hikes. Hearing the animals scurry through the woods, the crisp smell of the trees, and seeing the sun peeking through the clouds made me remember my purpose in life. This was what I needed to deal with my mental state. Nature has been my happy place as I struggle with depression on and off." - Alicia*

Spending time in nature helped this client through her depression. Being outdoors can do wonders for your overall health. Studies show that frequent exposure to greenspace (areas within an urban community covered with grass, trees, shrubs, and other vegetation) is associated with decreased levels of depression and loneliness. Surely there is somewhere in your vicinity where you can walk or hike. If it's a sunny day, you'll get an added bonus because the vitamin

D produced by the sunshine increases the production of serotonin, which is calming. You don't have to venture very far from home to enjoy the benefits of nature. Listening to chirping birds and taking notice of the plant life in your surroundings can be beneficial to your mental health. I am calmed when watching the ants and snails, or the clouds passing by. Another way to enjoy time outside is through a technique called grounding. Grounding focuses on direct or indirect contact with the earth by walking barefoot on grass, lying on the ground, or immersing in water. It is a way to help keep you in the present moment. As you immerse yourself in the natural world, you are boosting your physical and mental health. Based on numerous clinical studies, just spending 10 minutes outside can boost your mood. Although people commonly talk on their phones and listen to audiobooks, music, and podcasts while strolling, try walking without any extra auditory stimuli. Be alone with your thoughts and enjoy nature. If for some reason, you can't get outside, the simple step of sitting by a window may help you enjoy the sights in nature.

Other Therapies

<u>Laughter</u>

Have you ever heard any of these phrases, "laughter is the best medicine"; "laughter can be more satisfying than honor; more precious than money"? It is true – laughter is of great worth. Laughter can have a positive effect on conditions such as high blood pressure and heart disease and improve mental health. A few minutes of laughter can make us feel happier and more relaxed, which in turn helps us better handle the stressors of life. Children naturally laugh. I recently read that they do so at least 400 times a day. For adults, the estimate drops to a dismal daily count of 14. I strongly suggest you give this therapy a try and find ways to incorporate humor throughout your day. Take a few minutes to watch a funny video—Tik Tok, Instagram, and YouTube have lots of them. Spend time with friends and family that make you giggle.

Social Connection

Even though you may eat nutritious food, exercise regularly, get sufficient sleep, and receive medical treatment, you may still not feel well mentally. In these cases, it's important to consider what the cause may be. Might social isolation or feelings of "not belonging" be factors?

Human beings are wired for social connection. These connections are not just for entertainment or distraction—they improve mental health. Various studies show that social connections have health benefits including the reduction of stress, anxiety, and depression. To reap the benefits of these connections, strong relationships need to be formed with people you love and respect. Lack of social connection has the potential to not only cause anxiety, and depression, but has also been linked to earlier death, heart disease, and substance abuse. It's important to invest the time and energy in your relations. Living in isolation is dangerous to your mental health. Here are some suggestions to stay connected: volunteer, take a class, attend church, join a meetup/ small interest group, and spend time with friends and loved ones.

Acupuncture

Acupuncture is a form of Traditional Chinese Medicine (TCM) used to treat the whole body – mental and physical. Acupuncture is a procedure in which tiny needles are inserted at specific points on the body. In TCM, acupuncture is used to improve the flow of qi (pronounced "chi") or vital energy throughout the body, which is believed to positively affect both physical and mental health. It can also help you with spiritual, emotional, and physical balance as well as management of pain and trauma. Acupuncture is most effective when treatment is received at least two to three times a week. It is unlikely that going once or twice a month will be beneficial.

Final Remarks

There are many other types of therapies useful for managing anxiety and depression that are not mentioned in this chapter, such as massage therapy, vagus nerve stimulation therapy and craniosacral therapy. There are also various products advertised on the internet for lessening anxiety such as a wearable anxiety reducer designed to reduce your heart rate. I don't know if these products work as advertised. What I do know is that the therapies mentioned in this chapter have been scientifically researched and shown to be effective for many people. I have experienced the benefit of many of these therapeutic approaches such as physical exercise, mental exercise, drawing, guided meditation, prayer, and mindful journaling. I was able to effectively manage one of the most challenging health issues in my life through staying active, stimulating my mind and being socially active. Take a walk in nature, journal, play with your children, grandchildren, or beloved dog, or socialize with a friend.

These are some of the wonderful activities that can help regulate the rhythm of your mind and help your overall mental health. Set aside 15-30 minutes a day to engage in an activity that is beneficial, relaxing, and enjoyable for you.

CHAPTER SIX

GENETICS

"True wealth is having your health"

— Anonymous

When it comes to family history of diseases or conditions, I often hear statements such as: *"My mother had diabetes and high blood pressure, so that is why I have it." "It runs in the family." "Everyone in my family has that fat gene."* Whether it's depression, obesity, hypertension, or diabetes, many people think their genes are at fault. Sometimes doctors even tell their patients that genes are to be blamed when they can't find any other explanation for a problem. But could it be that you not only inherited these "unlucky" genes from your ancestors, but also became afflicted with a certain disease or condition because of the food you eat? Despite popular belief, most diseases, conditions, and disorders are not primarily driven by genetics, and are not simply the result of "bad luck"; it is more likely that the influences of diet, lifestyle, environment, and other behavioral factors are to blame.

Around the turn of the twentieth century, we learned that our genes are determined at conception. The Human Genome Project mapped out the entire human genome, which is the complete set of DNA instructions. At the fundamental level, genes are segments of a double-stranded chemical called DNA. DNA provides the basic instructions for the body and is stored in the nucleus of every cell. At this same time, researchers discovered that we are predisposed to inherit or become susceptible to certain diseases or health disorders, such as depression and diabetes, based on our genetic makeup or DNA. Since this time, there have been several hundred studies that have examined the influence of genetics on the body's response to nutrition and mental health. Nutrition, lifestyle, condition of the microbiome, and exposure to environmental pollutants are all factors that form a very complex relationship with our genes. It is said that "genetics loads the gun, but lifestyle pulls the trigger." If we are predisposed or at risk for certain diseases, and make unhealthy lifestyle choices, then we may be fulfilling the destiny of our genes.

It is estimated that humans have between 20,000 and 25,000 genes. Humans are 99% genetically identical, regardless of age or race. However, each of us has genetic variations that makes us unique. Have you ever bought clothing with a tag stating: "Fabric has intentional flaws in order to make it unique"? These variations are similar. There are millions of genetic differences that create our individual genetic blueprint. It is these "intentional variations" that make us unique and explain why some of us develop certain diseases or respond to certain diets while others do not. Genetic variations can result in both positive and negative impact. For instance, while some variations can make you feel anxious or sensitive to certain foods (e.g., foods containing dairy, wheat or gluten), others can result in increased intelligence or elite athletic status. There are still other variations that can predict the risk toward deficiencies in certain vitamins, the risk of developing certain diseases, and the response to certain medications. These variations may even help explain how and why your health issues may be different from members of your family.

This client's story gives some insight into genetic variations and mental health:

> "I was probably 8 years old when I realized I was sad. My mother left my father without saying goodbye to him or the children. So, I lived with my grandma until I was 13 years old. My grandmother would sometime help me feel happy, but I

often realized it was still easy for me to get sad when we weren't doing something fun. After that I lived with my wicked stepfather and two sisters. During my teens the depression got worse with changing hormones, and it was debilitating. By the time I was in my twenties and thirties, the mood swings became even more drastic – I would stay up several nights doing everything, and then sleep for two days straight. Other times I would lay on the floor and couldn't even talk. Nobody really talked about depression in the early 1990's. I somehow felt doomed because of the genes I inherited from my grandparents and parents. My maternal and paternal grandparents were alcoholics. My grandmother and mother had bad depression, and my grandmother ended up taking her life before she was sixty years old. My dad might have been depressed but he self-medicated with alcohol. My brother also has depression, and might be bipolar, but he uses drugs and alcohol to cope with his issues. And finally, my sister had depression and was an alcoholic, and then walked in front of a moving train one day."- Debra

In this case, analysis of her DNA revealed that she inherited several genetic variations which may have led to alcoholism and depression. Years ago, the link between genetics and mental health disorders, like depression and bipolar, were not even considered. But with the remarkable advances in genetic sequencing technology, we can see our complete DNA make up and look for genetic variations. Research shows that by changing some of our day-to-day activities, lifestyle behaviors, and food choices which affect our genes, we can directly impact the development of mental health disorders, heart disease, obesity, and many types of cancers. Getting genetic testing is a great way to start learning about your genetic variations. Why? Because it can provide insight into why you feel the way you do, both mentally and physically.

Nutrigenomics

The interaction between nutrition and genes has led to the creation of the new and emerging field of nutrigenomics (also known as nutritional genomics). Nutrigenomics is an area of genetic research that determines how food influences and acts on your genes. It is used to evaluate how we metabolize, absorb, and utilize the vitamins and minerals we get from the foods and beverages we consume. The food we eat has its own unique set of compounds that gives our genes the nutrient information needed to create the proteins our bodies require to work properly. When we eat food like meat, eggs, fish or legumes, the protein is digested and broken down into amino acids which our genes use to carry out their various bodily functions. The genetic variations can then determine whether the amino acids that are created are working properly or at their full capacity.

Let's look at a couple examples of how genetic variations may influence certain vitamin and mineral levels in the body and affect mental health. We know that we get vitamin D from exposing our skin to the sun and from eating certain food. After there has been an intake of vitamin D, it is used to perform numerous processes in the body, such as activating genes to make proteins that enable the absorption of calcium from the food you eat. But what if the activation of vitamin D is not working correctly because you have a genetic variation that impedes this process? In this case, your body will not be efficient at utilizing the vitamin D you get from the sun or the food and beverages you consume. This form of genetic variation may result in a lower vitamin D level which in turn is associated with symptoms of depression and anxiety, as well as low bone mineral density, and osteoporosis in post-menopausal women.

Another genetic variation that can affect mental health is associated with vitamin B9 also known as folate. Researchers found that this variation results in reduced activity of an enzyme used to convert the vitamin B9 from the foods we consume into a form to be used immediately by the body. Reduction in folate production can lead to various health conditions such as Alzheimer's disease, depression, colon cancer, stroke, and chronic fatigue. This enzyme is also important for the formation of neurotransmitters such as serotonin, epinephrine, norepinephrine, and dopamine. If you have a genetic tendency that impairs the production of this enzyme, then you will either make too much or too little of these neurotransmitters. Individuals who do not produce enough of these key neurotransmitters may have depression and other mental health symptoms. Those who make too much of these chemicals may have high anxiety, depression, and insomnia.

Genetic variations associated with vitamin D and vitamin B9 are just two examples of how the food we eat influences and acts on our genes. There are several hundred other genetic variations that are potentially associated with depression and anxiety. These variations affect the rate at which neurotransmitters, including serotonin, dopamine and norepinephrine are broken down and excreted from the body. Depending on the levels of these neurotransmitters, someone with variations in these genes could have mental health disorders such as depression and anxiety.

From a nutrition perspective, proper diet can ensure we are getting enough nutrients to create the neurotransmitters that activate genes for better mental health. One way to do this is by consuming phytonutrients, which are natural components of plants. Phytonutrients not only can improve mental health, but they have also been found to boost the immune system, protect against cancers, and help the body rid itself of toxins. Rich sources of phytonutrients are found in both grains and beans. Consuming a variety of fruits and vegetables, especially those having deep, dark, and bright colors, will often provide the best source of phytonutrients. Leave the skins and peels on these fruits and vegetables—they are a great source of phytonutrients, too. Blueberries and beets are wonderful choices. Other examples of foods that activate genes include broccoli, kale, and green cabbage. They all contain a phytonutrient called sulforaphane. Research shows that sulforaphane can activate certain genes which lead to tremendous beneficial effects on various mental health disorders such as anxiety.

We cannot choose our genes, but we can surely influence them in some way by our food choices. Let's use an analogy from the card game "Crazy Eights." You can't change the cards you are dealt, but if you get a wild card, you can use it to change the suit of the other cards and improve your hand. In the same way, you can't change your genetic makeup, but you can support your genes and improve your health by making wise food choices. Your genes are not your destiny and the existence of multiple variations in your genes does not dictate the state of your health. It is worth taking the time to consider making the best food and life-style choices to activate our genes and transform our mental health.

Conclusion

"Those who believe that they will be successful are more likely to persist in their goal-seeking and are more likely to succeed."

— Bandura

Stigma about mental health disorders keeps many of us silent, but it's a struggle that should be taken seriously. There is no reason to feel shame over any mental disorder you may be experiencing. Addressing our mental health needs is critical. It's not a sign of weakness. It takes strength and courage to talk about our mental health.

We know that the food we consume nourishes our body and affects our mind. Healthy eating, including attention to gut health, in combination with proper sleep and exercise are all important parts of emotional well-being and useful in cultivating good mental health. However, the nutritional approaches and therapies presented in this book should never be used exclusively to treat a serious medical condition, nor should they replace medications or other treatment methods currently being used. Any change in medication or treatment should first be thoroughly discussed and evaluated by your health care provider.

The root cause of my anxiety remains unknown. The problem could have arisen due to a hormonal imbalance, chronic stress, or a genetic predisposition to anxiety. I wanted to find alternative ways and a long-term solution to manage my problem before turning to the use of anti-anxiety medication. This led me to seek help from a naturopathic doctor. I felt comfortable confiding in her and she became a trusted friend. She recommended natural approaches to my problem such as changing diet and reducing stress through meditation and acupuncture. I did not experience immediate improvement. Rather, my healing came gradually through many of the approaches mentioned in this book such as dietary changes, exercise in the forms of tennis and golf, dietary and herbal supplements, professional counseling, and genomic testing and interpretation based on my personal DNA data. This combination of treatments helped me manage my feelings of anxiety, particularly during times when symptoms were severe.

When it comes to your mental health, each day can bring a new set of challenges to overcome. There are varying triggers, risk factors, genetics, hormonal changes, and food intolerances to consider. You must personalize the management of your mental health and work a little bit every day on building your "mental muscle" just as you would if you wanted to build muscles in your body.

I urge you to be open to trying various interventions and therapies as you work to overcome any mental health challenges you are battling. Be patient—it takes time and will involve trial and error. The journey will be different for everyone, but it is your responsibility to make the effort. Monitor your progress and check your mental health barometer frequently. As you learn to successfully address and manage your mental health, your story may be the inspiration for someone else. I hope my story and the stories of other people shared in this book has helped you.

APPENDIX A:

HOW TO CHOOSE QUALITY SUPPLEMENTS

Most dietary and herbal supplements are regulated by the U.S. Food and Drug Administration (FDA), although not as strictly as medications and over-the-counter drugs. Given the limited FDA regulation, there are many companies selling inexpensive supplements that are filled with contaminants, fillers, and allergens. This creates a host of complications for individuals trying to find the right quality supplement. Here are some tips when searching for safe, high-quality, and effective nutritional supplement products.

Tips:

- Products should be free of fillers (wheat, corn, or starches), preservatives, binders, lactose, coloring agents, shellacs, and other allergens.

- Products should be backed by current scientific research to support using the active ingredients for the claim(s) they make regarding health benefits.

- Products should include a disclaimer if the product is not FDA approved.

- Manufacturers should indicate use of supplement standards from an outside certifying body or third-party analysis for independent verification of active ingredients and contaminants. There are independent third-party testing and certification agencies such as USP and NSF International that work with supplement companies to certify that these products contain what is on the label, and do not contain harmful ingredients.

- Products should be in a form that is easily absorbed and utilized by the human body.

This food mood journal is a simple and effective tool that helps you become attuned to the signals your body sends you. By tracking what you eat and drink, you may become aware of connections between your diet and mood. As you notice these links, you will become increasingly motivated to make dietary choices that are beneficial to you.

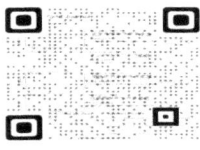 Scan the QR code to download the Food Journal

Amino acids – compounds that the body obtains from protein found in food

Antioxidants – molecules obtained from food which protect the cells from damage caused by free radicals.

Carbohydrates – sugar molecules found in foods

Cortisol – a hormone that is released in response to stress

Dopamine – a type of neurotransmitter released in the brain that is associated with pleasure, mood, and motivation

Endorphins – hormones that the brain releases in response to stress

Enzymes – substances that help speed up chemical reactions in the body

Estrogen – a hormone produced by the ovaries that plays a role in the sexual and reproductive health in women

Fermentation – a process in which bacteria and yeast breaks down sugar

Free radicals – molecules which can damage cells in the body

Hormones – natural chemicals produced by the body

Insulin – a hormone produced by the pancreas that helps remove excess sugar from the blood

Menopause – the time in life when a woman stops ovulating and menstruation ceases

Minerals – substances such as magnesium, calcium and potassium that are found in many foods

Microbiome – the collection of organisms (e.g., bacteria, fungi, and virus) living on the inside and outside of the body

Monosodium glutamate (MSG)– a widely used food additive contained in many commercial foods such as canned soups and vegetables to enhance flavor

Neurons – the fundamental units of the nervous system (also known nerve cells), which relay messages between the brain and nervous system

Neurotransmitters – chemicals that transmit information throughout the body

Norepinephrine – a type of neurotransmitter and hormone that is released in response to stress

Perimenopause – the time in a woman's life when gradual changes in the menstrual cycle begin, which eventually leads to menopause

Phytoestrogen – a compound which mimics estrogen that is derived from plants and can be found in various foods

Phytonutrients – natural compounds found in plant foods such as vegetables, fruit, legumes, and whole grain products

Psychotherapy – a treatment technique used by mental health professionals to help people with various mental health issues

Serotonin – a type of neurotransmitter associated with stabilizing and/or elevating mood

Testosterone – a sex hormone that regulates male sexual development

INDEX

A

alcohol, 11, 19, 26, 31, 33

amino acids, 29, 32, 70, 77

antioxidants, 29, 38, 40, 41, 42, 43, 49, 77

anxiety, 11

       triggers, 16, 17

       signs and symptoms, 15

anxiety disorders, 14

ashwagandha, 53

B

bacteria, 7, 22, 25, 27, 30, 40, 41, 42, 44, 46, 48

bananas, 41, 42, 52

B-Complex, 54

beneficial foods, 38, 40

blood sugar, 14, 30, 34, 46, 49, 51

blueberries, 42, 71

C

caffeine, 16, 29, 45, 46-48

cashews, 44, 52

chocolate, 43-44, 52

circadian rhythm, 36

CBT (cognitive behavioral therapy), 22

collard greens, 29, 42

cortisol, 13, 17, 33-35, 77

80

D

dairy, 35, 54, 69

depression, 18

> signs and symptoms, 20

depression disorders, 18

dopamine, 30, 43, 50, 58, 70, 71, 77

E

energy drinks, 47, 48

estrogen, 33, 34, 77

F

fiber, 29, 38, 40, 41, 42, 44, 49

food intolerance, 35-36

fruits, 32, 41-42, 46, 71

G

GAD (generalized anxiety disorder), 14

genes, 25, 36, 38, 44, 68-72

genetics, 19, 55, 68-72

gluten, 35-36, 68

green tea, 41, 45

H

heart disease, 6, 17, 64, 65, 69

herbal tea, 45

herbs, 38, 44, 54

hormonal imbalance, 33-34

hormones, 25, 33-34, 47, 51, 78

I

inflammation, 19, 35, 36, 38, 51

L

leafy greens, 42-43, 52

L-theanine, 45, 50

M

magnesium, 29, 42, 44, 49, 51-52

medications, 21-22

menopause, 16, 33

mental health, 6, 9

microbiome, 7, 25-27, 39, 41, 42, 46, 68, 78

minerals, 29, 32, 38, 40, 51, 70, 78

mushrooms, 43, 50

N

neurotransmitters, 24, 26, 29, 30-32, 41, 43, 44, 50, 54, 70-71, 78

non-medical therapies, 22, 56-66

nutrient deficiencies, 30-33, 49

nutrient-dense, 38, 39, 43

nutrigenomics, 7, 69-71

nutrition, 7, 29-29

nutritional psychiatry, 7, 29-30

nutritional therapy, 22-23

nuts, 33, 44, 51, 52

O

omega-3, 44, 49-51

P

phytonutrients, 38, 71, 79

prebiotics, 41

probiotics, 41, 49

problematic foods, 46

processed foods, 29, 32-33, 49

protein, 24, 29, 32-35, 39, 40, 44

psychotherapies, 22

pumpkin seeds, 33, 44, 52

S

seasonal affective disorder (SAD), 18

seeds, 33, 44, 51, 52

serotonin, 21, 22, 30, 42, 44, 45, 59, 64, 70, 71, 79

spices, 44

spinach, 39, 42

sugar, 11, 22, 32, 34-35, 39, 41, 46, 48, 49

sunflower seeds, 44

supplements, 49-55

T

testosterone, 33-34, 80

therapies, 56

        acupuncture, 65

        breathing, 61-62

        cooking, 57

        gardening, 57-58

        hobbies, 58

        journaling, 59

        laughter, 64

        meditation, 62

        mental exercises, 60-61

        music/calming sounds, 59

        nature, 63-64

        physical exercises, 60

        prayer, 62-63

        social connection, 65

trauma, 11, 14, 15, 66

V

vegetables, 29, 32, 42-43

vitamin B12, 50, 54-55

vitamin B6, 42, 54

vitamin B9, 54, 70, 71

vitamin C, 32, 55

vitamin D, 31-32, 45, 49, 52-53, 70

vitamins, 29, 31, 49, 54

W

walnuts, 44, 52

water, 45

ACKNOWLEDGMENTS

I cannot recall the moment the seeds were planted that would eventually become this book. As I reflect on the last sixty years of my life, my journey started in childhood, when my parents first placed the concept of health consciousness into my mind. My mother prepared breakfast every morning until I completed high school. At that time, I did not appreciate the importance of breakfast, but now I fully understand how critical it is to my behavior, thoughts, and mood. My father always had a garden filled with lots of fruits and vegetables, and he provided me with a great appreciation for home grown food—known today as organic food. I am very blessed and extremely grateful for my parents who established the foundation for healthy eating.

This year, 2022, was challenging for my entire family. With the loss of my father, I was not sure I wanted to or could continue writing this book. My husband, Duane, provided support, encouragement, and input to my numerous drafts. My sister, Andrea Moxam, championed my work from the very beginning. I owe a huge debt of gratitude to her for being my primary cheerleader. She believed in my ability to complete the book and encouraged me every day to keep writing. She also spent countless hours editing and providing critical feedback.

I am fortunate to have my best friend, Melinda Frankot, a retired speech/language pathologist, as my editor. I am thankful for the time she spent providing critical editorial comments and positive feedback. Every word matter and Melinda's guidance was taken seriously with each rewrite.

A huge heartfelt thanks goes out to my naturopathic doctor and mentor, Dr. Deborah Chelson. Dr. Chelson has been a huge supporter of my journey over the years to become a functional nutritionist, especially when I was pursuing my master's degree at the Maryland

University of Integrative Health. Dr. Chelson was also instrumental in helping me start my nutrition business. I am sincerely appreciative of her enthusiasm, expertise, and advice in health and nutrition.

Discussing mental health is often difficult. Many people do not know how or understand why nutrition plays a significant role in mental health disorders. I hope this book has made the subject relevant and easier to understand. My thanks to the women and men, who like me, have faced anxiety or depression and have been willing to share their stories.

Above all, I thank God for motivating me, guiding me, and providing me with the support team to complete this book.

Kathleen Gooden is the founder and owner of Gooden Healthy Nutrition, goodenhealthynutrition.com, specializing in functional nutrition counseling and genetics test interpretation. She holds a Master of Science degree in clinical nutrition and integrative health from the Maryland University of Integrative Health after previous work as a software developer. Between these two careers, she has accumulated 25 years of experience in problem-solving, and has developed interpersonal skills which enable her to effectively coach clients who are seeking improvements in their nutrition and lifestyle choices.

Kathleen passionately helps her clients understand the factors affecting their ability to obtain sustainable and healthy eating for life. She evaluates each client's health holistically, building their confidence and expanding their knowledge with healthy life choices. Kathleen conducts individualized nutritional interventions resulting in recommendations for improvement and behavior changes to afford the client optimal health.

Kathleen is a member of the American Nutrition Association. She is certified with Opus23 Explorer™ software, used for the analysis of genetics data, enabling her to interpret results from various nutrition-related genetic markers and to formulate nutritional plans. She also has a Mental Health First Aid (MHFA) certification that provides her with the training needed to recognize and respond to symptoms of mental health problems including depression, anxiety, and substance abuse disorders.

Kathleen is married to Duane, has four adult children, two grandchildren and a mixed terrier named Mickey. She currently resides in Arizona. She enjoys playing golf and tennis, drawing, walking her dog, and spending time with people who make her laugh.

ENDNOTES

Introduction

Mental health: Strengthening our response. (n.d.). Retrieved October 25, 2022, from https://www.who.int/news-room/fact-sheets/detail/mental-health-strengthening-our-response

Mental health awareness month 2022. (n.d.). Retrieved October 22, 2022, from National Council for Mental Wellbeing website: https://www.thenationalcouncil.org/mental-health-awareness-month/

Celano, C. M., Daunis, D. J., Lokko, H. N., Campbell, K. A., & Huffman, J. C. (2016). Anxiety disorders and cardiovascular disease. Current Psychiatry Reports, 18(11), 101. doi: 10.1007/s11920-016-0739-5

Chapter 1

Mental health awareness month 2022. (n.d.). Retrieved October 22, 2022, from National Council for Mental Wellbeing website: https://www.thenationalcouncil.org/mental-health-awareness-month/

Administration, S. A. and M. H. S. (2016, June). Table 3. 15, dsm-iv to dsm-5 generalized anxiety disorder comparison [Text]. Retrieved October 22, 2022, from https://www.ncbi.nlm.nih.gov/books/NBK519704/table/ch3.t15/

Celano, C. M., Daunis, D. J., Lokko, H. N., Campbell, K. A., & Huffman, J. C. (2016). Anxiety disorders and cardiovascular disease. Current Psychiatry Reports, 18(11), 101. doi: 10.1007/s11920-016-0739-5

Olafiranye, O., Jean-Louis, G., Zizi, F., Nunes, J., & Vincent, M. (2011). Anxiety and cardiovascular risk: Review of epidemiological and clinical evidence. Mind & Brain : The Journal of Psychiatry, 2(1), 32–37. Retrieved from https://www.ncbi.nlm.nih.gov/pmc/articles/PMC3150179/

Clarke, T. C., Schiller, J. S., & Boersma, P. (2020). Early release of selected estimates based on data from the 2019 national health interview survey. U.S. Department of Health and Human Services . Retrieved from https://www.cdc.gov/nchs/data/nhis/earlyrelease/EarlyRelease202009-508.pdf

Kirschner, H., Kuyken, W., & Karl, A. (2022). A biobehavioural approach to understand how mindfulness-based cognitive therapy reduces dispositional negative self-bias in recurrent depression. Mindfulness, 13(4), 928–941. doi: 10.1007/s12671-022-01845-3

Chapter 2

Valles-Colomer, M., Falony, G., Darzi, Y., Tigchelaar, E. F., Wang, J., Tito, R. Y., … Raes, J. (2019). The neuroactive potential of the human gut microbiota in quality of life and depression. Nature Microbiology, 4(4), 623–632. doi: 10.1038/s41564-018-0337-x

Perlmutter, David. (2017). Brain Maker: The Power of Gut Microbes to Heal and Protect Your Brain - for Life. (1st ed.). New York, NY: Little, Brown and Company.

Chapter 3

McCoy, C. R., Jackson, N. L., Brewer, R. L., Moughnyeh, M. M., Smith, D. L., & Clinton, S. M. (2018). A paternal methyl donor depleted diet leads to increased anxiety- and depression-like behavior in adult rat offspring. Bioscience Reports, 38(4), BSR20180730. doi: 10.1042/BSR20180730

Liu, J., Leung, P., & Yang, A. (2013). Breastfeeding and active bonding protects against children's internalizing behavior problems. Nutrients, 6(1), 76–89. https://doi.org/10.3390/nu6010076.

Shah, J., & Gurbani, S. (2019). Association of vitamin d deficiency and mood disorders: A systematic review. IntechOpen. doi: 10.5772/intechopen.90617

Lipski, E. (2012). Digestive wellness: Strengthen the immune system and prevent disease through healthy digestion (4th ed). New York, NY: McGraw-Hill.

Teufel, M., Biedermann, T., Rapps, N., Hausteiner, C., Henningsen, P., Enck, P., & Zipfel, S. (2007). Psychological burden of food allergy. World journal of gastroenterology, 13(25), 3456–3465. https://doi.org/10.3748/wjg.v13.i25.3456.

Manoogian, E. N. C., Chow, L. S., Taub, P. R., Laferrère, B., & Panda, S. (2021). Time-restricted eating for the prevention and management of metabolic diseases. Endocrine Reviews, 43(2), 405–436. doi: 10.1210/endrev/bnab027

Torquati, L., Mielke, G. I., Brown, W. J., Burton, N. W., & Kolbe-Alexander, T. L. (2019). Shift work and poor mental health: A meta-analysis of longitudinal studies. American Journal of Public Health, 109(11), e13–e20. doi: 10.2105/AJPH.2019.305278

Qian, J., Vujovic, N., Nguyen, H., Rahman, N., Heng, S. W., Amira, S., ... Chellappa, S. L. (2022). Daytime eating prevents mood vulnerability in night work. Proceedings of the National Academy of Sciences, 119(38), e2206348119. doi: 10.1073/pnas.2206348119

Chapter 4

LaChance, L. R., & Ramsey, D. (2018). Antidepressant foods: An evidence-based nutrient profiling system for depression. World Journal of Psychiatry, 8(3), 97–104. doi: 10.5498/wjp.v8.i3.97

Karbownik, M. S., Mokros, Ł., & Kowalczyk, E. (2022). Who benefits from fermented food consumption? A comparative analysis between psychiatrically ill and psychiatrically healthy medical students. International Journal of Environmental Research and Public Health, 19(7), 3861. doi: 10.3390/ijerph19073861

Głąbska, D., Guzek, D., Groele, B., & Gutkowska, K. (2020). Fruit and vegetable intake and mental health in adults: A systematic review. Nutrients, 12(1), 115. doi: 10.3390/nu12010115

Ba, D. M., Gao, X., Al-Shaar, L., Muscat, J. E., Chinchilli, V. M., Beelman, R. B., & Richie, J. P. (2021). Mushroom intake and depression: A population-based study using data from the US National Health and Nutrition Examination Survey (Nhanes), 2005-2016. Journal of Affective Disorders, 294, 686–692. doi: 10.1016/j.jad.2021.07.080

Shin, J.-H., Kim, C.-S., Cha, L., Kim, S., Lee, S., Chae, S., ... Shin, D.-M. (2022). Consumption of 85% cocoa dark chocolate improves mood in association with gut microbial changes in healthy adults: A randomized controlled trial. The Journal of Nutritional Biochemistry, 99, 108854. doi: 10.1016/j.jnutbio.2021.108854

Arab, L., Guo, R., & Elashoff, D. (2019). Lower depression scores among walnut consumers in nhanes. Nutrients, 11(2), E275. doi: 10.3390/nu11020275

Ramaholimihaso, T., Bouazzaoui, F., & Kaladjian, A. (2020). Curcumin in depression: Potential mechanisms of action and current evidence—a narrative review. Frontiers in Psychiatry, 11, 572533. doi: 10.3389/fpsyt.2020.572533

Knüppel, A., Shipley, M. J., Llewellyn, C. H., & Brunner, E. J. (2017). Sugar intake from sweet food and beverages, common mental disorder and depression: Prospective findings from the Whitehall II study. Scientific Reports, 7(1), 6287. doi: 10.1038/s41598-017-05649-7

Wang, W., Nettleton, J. E., Gänzle, M. G., & Reimer, R. A. (2022). A metagenomics investigation of intergenerational effects of non-nutritive sweeteners on gut microbiome. Frontiers in Nutrition, 8. Retrieved from https://www.frontiersin.org/articles/10.3389/fnut.2021.795848

Nca releases 2020 national coffee data trends, the "atlas of american coffee." (n.d.). Retrieved January 22, 2023, from https://www.ncausa.org/newsroom/nca-releases-atlas-of-american-coffee

Hidese, S., Ogawa, S., Ota, M., Ishida, I., Yasukawa, Z., Ozeki, M., & Kunugi, H. (2019). Effects of l-theanine administration on stress-related symptoms and cognitive functions in healthy adults: A randomized controlled trial. Nutrients, 11(10), E2362. doi: 10.3390/nu11102362

Kiecolt-Glaser, J. K., Belury, M. A., Andridge, R., Malarkey, W. B., & Glaser, R. (2011). Omega-3 supplementation lowers inflammation and anxiety in medical students: A randomized controlled trial. Brain, Behavior, and Immunity, 25(8), 1725–1734. doi: 10.1016/j.bbi.2011.07.229

Omega-3 fatty acids ease depressive symptoms related to menopause. (n.d.). Retrieved October 25, 2022, from ScienceDaily website: https://www.sciencedaily.com/releases/2009/01/090128104702.htm

Tarleton, E. K., Kennedy, A. G., Rose, G. L., Crocker, A., & Littenberg, B. (2019). The association between serum magnesium levels and depression in an adult primary care population. Nutrients, 11(7), 1475. doi: 10.3390/nu11071475

Botturi, A., Ciappolino, V., Delvecchio, G., Boscutti, A., Viscardi, B., & Brambilla, P. (2020). The role and the effect of magnesium in mental disorders: A systematic review. Nutrients, 12(6), 1661. doi: 10.3390/nu12061661

Pratte, M. A., Nanavati, K. B., Young, V., & Morley, C. P. (2014). An alternative treatment for anxiety: A systematic review of human trial results reported for the ayurvedic herb ashwagandha (Withania somnifera). Journal of Alternative and Complementary Medicine, 20(12), 901–908. doi: 10.1089/acm.2014.0177

Abdou, A. M., Higashiguchi, S., Horie, K., Kim, M., Hatta, H., & Yokogoshi, H. (2006). Relaxation and immunity enhancement effects of gamma-aminobutyric acid (Gaba) administration in humans. BioFactors (Oxford, England), 26(3), 201–208. doi: 10.1002/biof.5520260305

Sahraian, A., Ghanizadeh, A., & Kazemeini, F. (2015). Vitamin C as an adjuvant for treating major depressive disorder and suicidal behavior, a randomized placebo-controlled clinical trial. Trials, 16, 94. doi: 10.1186/s13063-015-0609-1

Chapter 5

Haley, L., & McKay, E. A. (2004). 'Baking gives you confidence': Users' views of engaging in the occupation of baking. British Journal of Occupational Therapy, 67(3), 125–128. doi: 10.1177/030802260406700305

J. W., & Nunnelley, P. A. (2016). Private prayer associations with depression, anxiety and other health conditions: An analytical review of clinical studies. Postgraduate Medicine, 128(7), 635–641. doi: 10.1080/00325481.2016.1209962

Fancourt, D., Opher, S., & de Oliveira, C. (2020). Fixed-effects analyses of time-varying associations between hobbies and depression in a longitudinal cohort study: Support for social prescribing? Psychotherapy and Psychosomatics, 89(2), 111–113. doi: 10.1159/000503571

Thoma, M. V., Marca, R. L., Brönnimann, R., Finkel, L., Ehlert, U., & Nater, U. M. (2013). The effect of music on the human stress response. PLOS ONE, 8(8), e70156. doi: 10.1371/journal.pone.0070156

Iodice, J. A. (2021). The association between gratitude and depression: A meta-analysis. International Journal of Depression and Anxiety, 4(1), 024. doi: 10.23937/2643-4059/1710024

Chapter 6

Anderson, J. W., & Nunnelley, P. A. (2016). Private prayer associations with depression, anxiety and other health conditions: An analytical review of clinical studies. Postgraduate Medicine, 128(7), 635–641. doi: 10.1080/00325481.2016.1209962

Bratman, G. N., Hamilton, J. P., Hahn, K. S., Daily, G. C., & Gross, J. J. (2015). Nature experience reduces rumination and subgenual prefrontal cortex activation. Proceedings of the National Academy of Sciences, 112(28), 8567–8572. doi: 10.1073/pnas.1510459112

Debusk, R. M., Fogarty, C. P., Ordovas, J. M., & Kornman, K. S. (2005). Nutritional genomics in practice: Where do we begin? Journal of the American Dietetic Association, 105(4), 589–598. doi: 10.1016/j.jada.2005.01.002

Liao, J. L., Qin, Q., Zhou, Y. S., Ma, R. P., Zhou, H. C., Gu, M. R., … Yang, L. (2020). Vitamin D receptor Bsm I polymorphism and osteoporosis risk in postmenopausal women: A meta-analysis from 42 studies. Genes & Nutrition, 15(1), 20. doi: 10.1186/s12263-020-00679-9

Moll, S., & Varga, E. A. (2015). Homocysteine and mthfr mutations. Circulation, 132(1), e6–e9. doi: 10.1161/CIRCULATIONAHA.114.013311

Zhang, J.-C., Yao, W., Dong, C., Yang, C., Ren, Q., Ma, M., … Hashimoto, K. (2017). Prophylactic effects of sulforaphane on depression-like behavior and dendritic changes in mice after inflammation. The Journal of Nutritional Biochemistry, 39, 134–144. doi: 10.1016/j.jnutbio.2016.10.004

Ferreira-Chamorro, P., Redondo, A., Riego, G., Leánez, S., & Pol, O. (2018). Sulforaphane inhibited the nociceptive responses, anxiety- and depressive-like behaviors associated with neuropathic pain and improved the anti-allodynic effects of morphine in mice. Frontiers in Pharmacology, 9, 1332. doi: 10.3389/fphar.2018.01332